EMERGENCY MEDICAL SERVICES FOR CHILDREN: THE ROLE OF THE PRIMARY CARE PROVIDER

Author:
Committee on Pediatric Emergency Medicine
American Academy of Pediatrics

Jonathan Singer, MD, Editor
Stephen Ludwig, MD, Associate Editor

American Academy of Pediatrics
141 Northwest Point Blvd
PO Box 927
Elk Grove Village, IL 60009-0927

Library of Congress Catalog No. 92-73819

ISBN No. 0-910761-37-X

Quantity prices on request. Address all inquiries to:
American Academy of Pediatrics
141 Northwest Point Blvd, PO Box 927
Elk Grove Village, IL 60009-0927

COMMITTEE ON PEDIATRIC EMERGENCY MEDICINE 1991-1992

Stephen Ludwig, MD, Chairperson, 1988-1992
J. Alexander Haller, Jr, MD
Marc L. Holbrook, MD
Jane Knapp, MD
William J. Lewander, MD
James S. Seidel, MD, PhD
Calvin C.J. Sia, MD
Jonathan Singer, MD
Joseph A. Weinberg, MD

Liaison Representatives

Max L. Ramenofsky, MD
American College of Surgeons

Robert W. Schafermeyer, MD
American College of Emergency Physicians

AAP Section Liaisons

Daniel Notterman, MD
Section on Critical Care

James O'Neill, MD
Section on Surgery

Staff

Susan M. Tellez

ACKNOWLEDGMENTS

The Committee gratefully acknowledges the following persons who are not Committee members who contributed initial drafts for some chapters.

George L. Foltin, MD, FAAP
Bellevue Hospital Center
New York, NY

Robert C. Luten, MD, FAAP
University Hospital of Jacksonville
Jacksonville, FL

Karin A. McCloskey, MD, FAAP
University of Alabama at Birmingham
Birmingham, AL

Richard A. Orr, MD, FAAP
Children's Hospital at Pittsburgh
Pittsburgh, PA

Joseph E. Simon, MD, FAAP
Scottish Rite Children's Medical Center
Atlanta, GA

Michael G. Tunik, MD, FAAP
Bellevue Hospital Center
New York, NY

EMERGENCY MEDICAL SERVICES FOR CHILDREN: THE ROLE OF THE PRIMARY CARE PROVIDER

COMMITTEE ON PEDIATRIC EMERGENCY MEDICINE

TABLE OF CONTENTS

Appendix

Tables

PREFACE

Almost 15 years ago, a small group of physicians who were working in the pediatric emergency departments came to the American Academy of Pediatrics to ask what might be done to improve the care of children who were suffering acute illness or injury. The Academy generously gave us a home in the Ad Hoc Section of Pediatric Emergency Medicine. Allowing us to meet regularly, share ideas, and dream our dreams was a critically important step in working toward improving child health and emergency care.

The ad hoc section grew into a regular standing section, which now has nearly 500 members. The Academy also encouraged the formation of a Committee on Pediatric Emergency Medicine (COPEM). In 1988 we published a simple statement of our intent: "Pediatrician's Role in Emergency Medical Services for Children" (see Appendix A). A great deal of activity has taken place since.

There have been official ties formed with other AAP sections, including Pediatric Surgery and Critical Care; with other organizations such as the American College of Surgeons, the American Society of Pediatric Surgeons, the American College of Emergency Physicians, the Society for Pediatric Emergency Medicine, and the Ambulatory Pediatric Association.

In developing a system of emergency care for children, we have worked in several arenas. We have developed the specialty of Pediatric Emergency Medicine now approved by the American Board of Pediatrics and the American Board of Emergency Medicine. The first board-certification examination is scheduled for November 1992.

The body of knowledge of pediatric emergency medicine has been codified by many books, manuals, and monographs. Fellowship programs have been established to encourage young people to make a career commitment to pediatric emergency medicine. Courses such as Pediatric Advanced Life Support (PALS) and Advanced Pediatric Life

Support (APLS) have been offered to upgrade the knowledge and skills of the practicing primary care provider. In addition, we have done extensive work to improve the knowledge, skills, and attitudes of prehospital care providers. The federal government, through Emergency Medical Services System for Children (EMS-C) grants, has encouraged states to improve EMS-C. The funding for these grants has had the dedicated stewardship of Senator Daniel K. Inouye of Hawaii. The products of the grants are available for all of us to use (see Appendices B and C).

This manual represents an expansion of the 1988 statement. It is an attempt to encourage each of the 44,000 members of the Academy and each primary care provider to get involved, to become part of the EMS-C. The moment of a true emergency is a critical point in a child's life and in the life of his or her family. Not unlike the moment of birth, an emergency is pivotal to the chance for continued life and all that it offers, or the despair and loss that accompanies the death of a child or the loss of his or her intactness. Good emergency care makes a difference. As primary care providers we want to feel that we have done the best that we can do. We want to make a difference. It is our hope that each and every primary care provider will read through this volume and make changes that will improve the emergency care of children. On behalf of the children of our country and my COPEM colleagues, I thank you for doing so.

Stephen Ludwig, MD
Chairperson
Committee on Pediatric
Emergency Medicine

September 1992

CHAPTER 1

THE PRIMARY CARE PROVIDER'S ROLE IN EMS-C

Are you a part of the "system"?

What "system," you ask?

The Emergency Medical Services System for Children—the EMS-C.

Whether you know it or not, *you* are an important part of the EMS-C. When one hears the term EMS-C, Emergency Medical Services for Children, thoughts of emergency departments, ambulances, paramedics, and intensive care units come to mind. Figure 1 and Table 1 offer an example of a conceptual framework for an EMS-C and a listing of its components. Office- and clinic-based primary care providers are critically important elements in the emergency care system for children. This manual will be helpful to primary care providers in reevaluating their many special roles in delivering emergency care to children. Even if all the emergency departments, intensive care units, and ambulances in the United States were at the highest level of functioning, we would still need the primary care providers' efforts to have a system capable of saving lives. The EMS-C is a multidisciplinary system for providing care. It includes you.

What are the primary care provider's roles in EMS-C? This manual is intended to answer that question. Obviously there are many roles. To highlight a few, they include educator, triage officer, emergency care provider, consultant, child advocate, and disaster coordinator. Primary care providers must realize what they can do as part of the EMS-C system.

EMS-C: An Integrated System

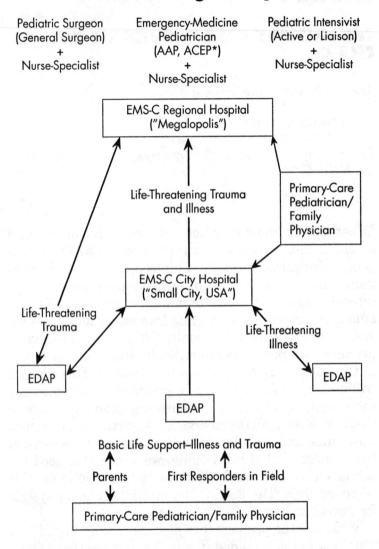

Pediatric Surgeon (General Surgeon) + Nurse-Specialist

Emergency-Medicine Pediatrician (AAP, ACEP*) + Nurse-Specialist

Pediatric Intensivist (Active or Liaison) + Nurse-Specialist

EMS-C Regional Hospital ("Megalopolis")

Life-Threatening Trauma and Illness

Primary-Care Pediatrician/ Family Physician

EMS-C City Hospital ("Small City, USA")

Life-Threatening Trauma

Life-Threatening Illness

EDAP

EDAP

EDAP

Basic Life Support–Illness and Trauma

Parents   First Responders in Field

Primary-Care Pediatrician/Family Physician

*AAP = American Academy of Pediatrics
ACEP = American College of Emergency Physicians

Fig 1. EMS-C: An Integrated System. From Haller JA. 97th Ross Conference. Ross Laboratories, 1989.

Table 1. — Components of a Comprehensive EMS-C System.*

I. Patient education, anticipatory prevention, injury control by pediatrician/family physician

II. Modes of entry—formally identified
   A. Physician's office
   B. Parents (911 telephone system)
   C. Health maintenance organization
   D. Community emergency rooms (ERs), including emergency departments approved for pediatrics (EDAPs)

III. Emergency medical technicians (EMTs) and paramedics—physician supervision
   A. On-line control
   B. Field protocols

IV. Communication
   A. Via emergency-medicine communication center (EMCC)
      1. To designated EMS-C center
      2. To on-line responder
         a. Emergency-medicine pediatrician
         b. Pediatric nurse-specialist
   B. Physician to physician
      1. ER physician to responsible physician in EMS-C hospital (interhospital)

V. Acute stabilization of patient in appropriate resuscitation center (EDAP)
   A. Airway
   B. Breathing
   C. Circulation

VI. Transport
   A. Air or ground via EMCC
      1. On-line input from EMS-C physician

VII. Patient management at designated EMS-C center
   A. Responsibilities
      1. Internal management protocols
      2. Quality assurance
      3. Regular morbidity and mortality conferences
   B. Functions
      1. Evaluation
      2. Resuscitation
      3. Extended diagnosis
   C. Composite care team
      1. Leader: Physician most experienced in child's primary condition

Table 1. — Components of a Comprehensive EMS-C System.* (continued)

    a. Trauma: usually pediatric surgeon
    b. Illness: usually emergency-medicine pediatrician
 2. Members of EMS-C team
    a. Pediatric general surgeon
    b. Pediatric specialty surgeon
       (eg, orthopedic, neurologic)
    c. Emergency-medicine pediatrician (American Academy of
       Pediatrics or American College of Emergency
       Physicians)
    d. Pediatric nurse-specialists
    e. Pediatric intensivist or anesthesiologist
    f. Primary pediatrician (for liaison with family and continuity
       of care)

VIII. Pediatric intensive care: Composite team[†]
   A. Leader
      1. Determined by team
      2. Most experienced physician in primary condition
         a. eg, Pediatric intensivist for near-drowning victim

 IX. Intermediate (step-down) care[†]
   A. Management leadership decided by primary-condition
      physician

  X. Rehabilitation
   A. Types
      1. Physical
      2. Psychologic
      3. Dental
   B. Leadership: Best-qualified person identified
      by care team

 XI. Patient release and follow-up by primary-care pediatrician/family
     physician

XII. Patient-data surveillance (in-line monthly review, off-line
     quarterly reports)
   A. Results of rehabilitation
   B. Final status

---

*Adapted from Haller JA. 97th Ross Conference. Ross Laboratories, 1989. This Comprehensive Emergency Medical Services for Children (EMS-C) Systems Components outline illustrates the proposed sequence of a child's/parent's utilization of components of an EMS-C system from anticipatory prevention to full rehabilitation and return to home and family. The precise organization of each of the components will depend on local and regional resources, and the final system must be derived locally by all pediatric medical and paramedical personnel who are committed to the care of seriously ill and injured children.

†Whenever appropriate, the primary care provider should be involved if on staff.

Educator

The primary care provider often serves in the role of educator. The most important educational message is that of prevention. Prevention of potential emergency conditions is ultimately the most effective treatment strategy. Beyond trying to thwart emergency situations, the primary care provider must educate the patient and parents about their response to emergencies. When to call the office versus when to go directly to the emergency department (ED)? Which is the best hospital to select? When should a parent drive to the ED as opposed to calling for paramedics? How does one obtain access to the local ambulance company? What should be done while the child is at the babysitter's? These and many other questions need to be asked and answered by the primary care provider. Also, all parents should be encouraged to take instruction in basic life support (CPR) through the American Heart Association or the American Red Cross.

Triage Officer

As a triage officer, the primary care provider and the office staff must be prepared to direct families to the nearest emergency care center that is fully capable in managing childhood emergencies. A hospital that posts an Emergency Department sign over its door does not always guarantee optimal pediatric emergency care. Some patients are safe to wait until tomorrow's office hours, some must be seen immediately.

Emergency Care Provider

There will be situations in which the primary care provider must be the direct provider of emergency care. In this role the primary care provider must have the correct combination of knowledge, technical skills, and attitudes to get the job done. It is also critical to have the proper equipment and preparation of office staff to react to an emergency situation. There now exists the possibility to gain this training through the Pediatric Advanced Life Support and Advanced Pediatric Life Support courses. This manual will present lists of suggested office equipment and address other issues of office preparedness. Studies have shown that many primary care providers do not have basic life support equipment in their offices and that many may not have an organized plan for safely transporting a critically ill child from the office to the hospital.

Consultant/Child Advocate

In the role of consultant and child advocate, the primary care provider must know what is the state of the local community hospital ED and the local transport or ambulance system in regard to emergency care of pediatric patients. Many will be horrified to find a lack of equipment, training, or mind-set to really take care of an ill or injured child. Primary care providers can advocate for their patients so that these deficiencies may be corrected. The pediatric emergency training of many otherwise well-qualified emergency physicians has not been what it should be.

Disaster Management

Imagine what would happen in your community if there were a mass casualty situation involving a significant number of children. Is your community prepared? Do the primary care providers have a disaster plan? Is there an emergency telephone tree that could serve to alert everyone? What is the state AAP chapter doing to foster training in emergency care?

Summary

This manual will familiarize you with EMS-C and how you can become a more active "player" in the system. It will offer case scenarios to set the stage, a glossary of equipment terms, practical information, and action steps that you can take. The most important function that this manual can serve is to bring you and your pediatric, emergency medicine, surgical, paramedic, and nursing colleagues together to consider what can be done in your community. Emergency care of children is everyone's concern.

As primary care providers, we have a huge role to carry out if we are to reduce the morbidity and mortality of childhood. Many life-threatening situations offer a window of opportunity to save a life or at least to lessen the impact of an illness or injury. We have the knowledge and the skills. We need the interest, the mind-set, the cooperation, and the determination to make a difference.

Bibliography

1. Foltin G, Fuchs S. Advances in pediatric emergency medical service systems. *Emerg Med Clin North Am*. 1991;9:459-474

2. Haller JA, ed. *Emergency Medical Services for Children: Report of the 97th Ross Conference on Pediatric Research*. Columbus, OH: Ross Laboratories, 1989:1-145

3. Ludwig S, Selbst S. A child-oriented emergency medical services system. *Curr Probl Pediatr*. 1990;20:109-158

CHAPTER 2

WHAT IS EMS-C AND WHERE DOES THE PRIMARY CARE PHYSICIAN FIT IN?

Cases

A 6-year-old boy falls a distance of 6 ft off the jungle gym in his backyard onto his right shoulder.

A 13-year-old girl faints at school.

A 4-year-old boy is hit by a car after darting into the street while playing tag.

A 2-year-old ingests two of grandpa's "heart pills."

One of your patients may become suddenly ill or injured, perhaps at home, perhaps at school, or while at play. Unexpectedly, a child is in need of emergency care. The families you care for have probably given very little thought as to how they will have access to this care. In all likelihood they assume a system is in place.

Question

Is there a system in place to deliver appropriate emergency care to your pediatric patients in your community?

Key Terms

Key terms in EMS-C are listed here and in Appendix D.

Emergency Medical Service (EMS) System: A group of organizations that collectively provide emergency care to acutely ill or injured persons.

Emergency Medical Service System for Children (EMS-C): Describes the broad-based effort to provide emergency care for the acutely ill or injured child.

911: A telephone system that provides direct access to an EMS system; activation triggers a coordinated and medically directed ambulance, fire, and/or police dispatch.

Enhanced 911: A telephone-based system in which activation provides a dispatcher information regarding location of all calls, enabling a link to emergency systems by persons unable to communicate the exact address and phone number of a call, including young children.

Sudden illness and injury described in the above scenarios have the following in common.

1. They are largely preventable, but when they occur, they are often reversible if treated appropriately in a timely manner.

2. They are acute/emergent in presentation and often occur without prior warning. Frequently the occurrence represents the most acute and critical period of physiologic derangements (eg, seizures), or represents the initiation of a critical time period in which intervention must occur if treatment is to be successful.

3. In the most acute phase of the disease process, patients are frequently attended by a provider lacking specialization in the care of a particular disease entity. In most instances, the provider with the most expertise and experience in the given disease process is the furthest removed in the hierarchy of health care and may have little or no input into management protocols utilized by the first responder to these emergency conditions.

Before the primary care provider can answer the question concerning medical systems in his or her own community, it is vital to have an understanding of the EMS system. The term EMS system refers to a group of distinct health care delivery organizations that, when taken together, allow for the appropriate delivery of care to the suddenly ill or injured. The federal government has taken the position since the early 1970s that these diverse services be considered together in a functioning EMS system designed to deliver care. The following is an overview of the development and components of an intact EMS system.

Historically, EMS systems formed in the 1970s. Priorities at that time were adult trauma and cardiac disease. Significant strides have been made in these areas with the use of advanced cardiac life support techniques for adults and the creation of trauma centers and trauma systems.

The founders of EMS systems were trained in adult specialties and worked with little input from the pediatric community. It is not surprising that the special needs of children were not considered within an adult-oriented EMS system. Children make up less than 10% of prehospital ambulance runs and less than 1% of the critically ill patients. Only recently has attention turned to the needs of children in the EMS system, and it has been shown that there is work to be done if those needs are to be met.

The specialty referral component of the EMS Act of 1973 addressed the need to regionalize seven target populations within the EMS system. These included patients with cardiac problems, trauma, burns, spinal cord injuries, behavioral emergencies, poisoning, and neonatal care, but the measure did not address the issues regarding regionalization of care for the critically ill and injured pediatric patient.

Of interest, the community concerned with neonatal care pioneered concepts of regionalization, categorization, and transport for a civilian setting for the unique population they treat.

Within the various components of an intact EMS system are contained all the elements commonly agreed upon as being essential for an EMS system. Those discussed in this chapter are medical direction, prehospital transport agencies, dispatch, communications, protocols (prehospital triage, prehospital treatment, transport, and transfer), receiving facilities, specialty care units, quality assurance, and public education. Other important elements are disaster management (Chapter 9) and interfacility transport agencies (Chapter 7). These essential elements were outlined in the EMS Act of 1973 (PL-154) which, as previously mentioned, spurred the growth of EMS nationally in the 1970s.

The following components are ways to conceive of an intact EMS system.

1. **Access and system entry:** This consists of patient and citizen education on (1) prevention, (2) bystander CPR and obstructed airway training, (3) recognition of the critical medical conditions such as seizures and signs of cardiac and severe respiratory impairment such as choking and apnea, as well as (4) how to gain access to the local emergency response system, which should be a 911 system, and optimally is an enhanced 911 system. Once 911 has been activated, trained personnel then perform telephone triage to dispatch the appropriate or available level of emergency response.

2. **Prehospital care:** This includes first response and transport by basic emergency medical technicians and paramedics, as well as by police and fire department personnel (Chapter 5). Within this framework are triage decisions for specialty referrals such as trauma center candidates, and provision of in-field basic life support and advanced life support treatment utilizing protocols. This specialized medical care is delivered under the umbrella of direct (on-line) and indirect (off-line) medical control.

   Indirect medical control consists of the physician input into the creation and ongoing maintenance of the prehospital component of EMS. A medical director, or medical advisory committee, takes responsibility for developing triage and treatment guidelines for prehospital providers as well as for developing educational programs. They also provide quality assurance for the system.

Direct medical control consists of direct contact between prehospital personnel and a physician. This may occur via radio or telephone. Usually the physician giving direct medical control will provide medical guidance as developed and limited by indirect medical control. By remaining within medical guidelines approved by the medical community, liability is limited for the prehospital providers and the physician providing the direct medical control. Most systems have base stations set up in emergency departments where an on-duty emergency physician will provide the direct medical control in addition to his or her regular duties. Some systems with a large enough patient volume will have physicians dedicated solely to this task.

Field triage allows patients to be directed to the appropriate facility to meet their emergent needs. Prehospital personnel will sort patients using predetermined criteria or direct medical control. The trauma center concept cannot exist without this sorting to bring the more severely injured patients to the trauma centers and less acutely injured patients to nontrauma centers. Very few systems sort children for trauma or medical problems.

3. **In-hospital emergency care:** This includes categorization and designation of institutions to identify the level of care that an institution is capable of delivering. An individual institution's capabilities may differ in the delivery of different services. The American Medical Association's Commission on Emergency Medical Services advocated this horizontal classification of emergency services by defining varying levels of care for ten different areas, including trauma, burns, cardiology, and pediatrics. Although trauma center systems have been demonstrated to improve outcome, their successful implementation, nationwide, is far from complete. A

recent report from the National Highway Traffic Safety Administration noted that currently only 21 states have an active trauma center program, with many of these lacking integration of prehospital services with the trauma center system.

Victims of trauma in rural settings face a special challenge. Certain factors in rural trauma, such as large, sparsely populated areas that EMS systems must cover, result in special problems. A compounding problem is that severe trauma occurs infrequently in any given location in the rural setting. Rural prehospital and hospital staff will be called upon to assess and stabilize patients with injuries *as severe* as their urban counterparts, but on an infrequent basis. Surprisingly, 70% of all highway fatalities occur on rural roads. Pediatric victims of severe rural trauma clearly are an especially high-risk group.

4. **Definitive care:** Following resuscitation and stabilization, children may require further definitive care. Certain patients may require an operative procedure. Certain patients may require care in a pediatric intensive care unit. The victim of trauma may require a laparotomy to control hemorrhage, a pin to put a femur fracture under traction, or a craniotomy for an intracerebral hemorrhage. The majority of severely injured children will have non-operative injuries but still require the attention of pediatric surgeons, pediatric intensivists, pediatric nurses, and a pediatric intensive care unit. Severe head injuries may require intracranial pressure monitoring and the involvement of a neurosurgeon for appropriate management. A severely ill patient may require resuscitation in the emergency department and, subsequently, continued treatment in the pediatric intensive care unit. If an institution is not

capable of delivering definitive care, does it have a transfer system that works in a timely manner?

5. **Rehabilitation:** This really begins at the moment the patient enters the acute care system. It is a crucial component requiring planning, facilities, and staff to ensure a favorable outcome.

When the various components of the EMS system and the essential elements that are associated with each one are examined, we see that the EMS system does not fall under the aegis of any one organization, agency, or specialty group. These components are often operating independently, may not interface well or at all with the other components, or may not exist at all. This varies on a region-to-region basis. The needs of children have not been adequately addressed in the EMS system and are different in each of the components. The pediatric challenge of an effective EMS system has to be met on many different levels and in a variety of settings.

Emergency medical services for children is a broad-based effort to incorporate appropriate health care delivery to suddenly ill or injured children into an already existing adult-oriented EMS system. The federal government has manifested interest in this effort by funding EMS-C demonstration grants since 1985, with the majority of states having been funded. The goals of this EMS-C project are (1) to reduce sequelae of pediatric emergencies at state and local levels, (2) to generate financial support for continuation of EMS-C programs after federal support terminates, and (3) to aid neighboring states to develop programs to meet these goals.

The primary care provider has an important role in working to improve emergency medical services for children. One role is educating parents and other caretakers (Chapter 3). Teaching such skills as recognition of significant illness or injury, how and when to access appropriate levels of care, and where to obtain training in CPR are all forms of anticipatory guidance that should be taught by the primary care provider. A vital aspect of public education is prevention. Informed parents who take responsibility for the safety of their children, and safety-conscious children themselves, are keys to effective prevention. Public awareness efforts should be directed to this end, and primary care providers play a major role in this phase through parent education.

Action Points

1. Primary care providers can provide a unifying role in EMS-C. As envisioned by Calvin Sia, MD, a pediatrician from Hawaii, the physician may continue to care for an ill child throughout a critical event. The primary care provider may provide support to the child and family even if subspecialists at the referral center are temporarily providing definitive care. Once the acute phase has passed, the primary care provider would coordinate rehabilitative care with the goal of returning the child to the level of activity that was normal before the critical event occurred. This concept has been termed "the medical home" (Chapter 10).

2. Primary care physicians can educate themselves about optimal levels of hospital resources to render effective care. An important document outlining standards for care of children in hospitals has been prepared by the American Medical Association—Emergency Medical Service (AMA-EMS) Commission and published in *Pediatrics* by the American Academy of Pediatrics. The AMA-EMS classification guidelines (Appendix E) outline the staffing, equipment, and programs necessary for hospitals to deliver pediatric emergency care, designated as levels 1, 2, or 3. Primary care providers can compare these national guidelines to what is actually available in their area and work to improve the EMS-C system in their local environment.

3. Primary care physicians should work to improve all components of their local, regional, and state EMS systems. Perhaps the most crucial link is the establishment of a system to assure that critically ill or injured children will be cared for in a setting appropriate to their illness or injury. One of the longest running successful models for regionalization of care is the Maryland Institute of Emergency Medical Services Systems of Maryland and Washington, DC, where all significantly injured children are transported by helicopter or ground transport to a pediatric trauma center. Many regions of California have adopted a voluntary regionalization plan consisting of emergency departments appropriate for pediatrics and pediatric critical care centers. Other states such as Pennsylvania and New York have included pediatric trauma centers in their trauma center systems. It is imperative that the prehospital care providers recognize and utilize the programs that establish themselves as resource or referral centers for prehospital care of pediatric patients.

4. The primary care provider may promote the incorporation of EMS-C into preexisting EMS and may join a host of multidisciplined persons who can work together to integrate the system.

5. Primary care physicians should advocate for 911 or enhanced 911 systems.

AAP Resources

Luten R, Foltin G, eds. *Pediatric Resources for Prehospital Care*. Elk Grove Village, IL: American Academy of Pediatrics; 1990

Bibliography

American Medical Association Commission on Emergency Medical Services. Pediatric emergencies: an excerpt from "Guidelines for the Categorization of Hospital Emergency Capabilities." *Pediatrics.* 1990;85: 879-887

Barkin RM, ed. Pediatrics in the emergency medical services system. *Pediatr Emerg Care.* 1990;6:72-77

Foltin G, Salomon S, Tunik M, Schneiderman W, Treiber M. Developing prehospital advanced life support for children: the New York City experience. *Pediatr Emerg Care.* 1990;6: 141-144

Haller JA, ed. *Emergency Medical Services for Children: Report of the 97th Ross Conference on Pediatric Research.* Columbus, OH: Ross Laboratories; 1989: 1-145

National Highway Traffic Safety Administration. *Emergency Medical Services: 1990 and beyond.* Washington, DC: NHTSA; October 1990. US Dept of Transportation publication DOT HS 807 639

Seidel JS, Henderson DP, eds. Emergency Medical Services for Children: a report to the nation. National Center for Education in Maternal and Child Health, Washington, DC, 1991

CHAPTER 3

PREPARING PARENTS TO COPE WITH EMERGENCIES

Cases

A 16-month-old boy in the course of exploring the contents of his mother's purse is witnessed to swallow a coin. After transiently gagging, the child seems uncomfortable and is noted to drool excessively.

A 6-year-old girl, while running, chokes on a piece of hard candy. She cannot speak and coughs ineffectively. The parent performs a Heimlich maneuver, permitting the child to breathe again. After the event, the child complains of a sore throat.

A preadolescent with a known seizure disorder has a generalized tonic-clonic seizure after sustaining an apparently trivial head injury in a fall from a bicycle.

Questions

1. Have parents of these children received advice from their primary care providers in techniques of injury prevention?

2. Do these parents know that a potential emergency medical condition exists in their children?

3. What role does the primary care provider play in preparation of families for emergencies?

Key Terms

Basic Life Support (BLS): A responder to an emergency who has the capabilities to provide adequacy of airway, ventilation, and circulation.

Advanced Life Support (ALS): In addition to BLS capacity, this responder to an emergency can provide resuscitation drugs.

Parents must be educated from many different perspectives with respect to emergency medical conditions that may affect their children. These perspectives range from preventing emergency conditions to advocacy for appropriate community resources to deal with emergencies when they arise.

Prevention

The best solution to the problem presented by a child entering the Emergency Medical Services (EMS) system is to prevent the need for the child to enter the system in the first place. Therefore, effective injury prevention education is a key component of any comprehensive local or regional EMS system for children. Primary care providers have a key role to play in this component of the system through anticipatory guidance.

Anticipatory guidance can be performed in many ways. Direct physician-parent discussion of safety hazards and appropriate precautions at various ages has been shown to be of clear benefit. To be most effective, this anticipatory guidance should be tailored to the risks prevalent in a given community. Some form of community surveillance via local emergency facility statistics or by International Class of Disease-E coding (ICD-E) hospital discharges should be established. ICD-E coding systems classify external causes of injury, such as motor vehicle accident, in contrast to ICD-H coding systems that classify the nature of the injury, such as closed head injury. Identified trends can be made available to primary care providers and others involved in anticipatory guidance, injury prevention, and community health. This surveillance and the resulting anticipatory guidance should focus not just on accidental injury, but on the whole gambit of potentially preventable emergency conditions, including infectious diseases that may be prevented through immunization, improved hygiene, or reduced exposure risk, sexual abuse, psychological trauma, and ill-advised home remedies for minor illness.

Anticipatory guidance is a very time-consuming activity. At the 2-year checkup, for example, there are no fewer than 15 different injury risks to be potentially reviewed with the parent. Using a separate billing code for anticipatory guidance at certain ages might make the time spent more cost-effective for the primary care provider, particularly when coupled with lobbying efforts to obtain reimbursement for this code. Another approach is the TIPP program of the Academy. This program provides appropriate anticipatory guidance for each health supervision visit from birth to the age of 8 years.

Yet another approach would be to strongly encourage parents to take the CPR-Infant and Child course developed by the American Red Cross or the Pediatric BLS course developed by the AHA. While both courses teach CPR, both actually devote the majority of course time to injury and injury prevention. Both courses offer "hands-on" activity and testing resulting in excellent 6-month retention of the information provided. Another virtue of this approach to anticipatory guidance is that, unlike a visit to the office of the primary physician, both parents can be encouraged to participate under the guise of learning CPR. Finally, this approach provides the added reinforcement of peer pressure—other parents in the course who share their concerns and experiences with respect to injury prevention.

Some communities have dealt with the challenge of anticipatory guidance using the mass media. A talk show involving primary care providers is one possible format. Another format might include public service radio and television announcements. A third possibility is to form a contact with the medical writer of a local newspaper or magazine.

Anticipatory guidance involves educating parents in techniques of "active" injury prevention—techniques that involve at least one action on the part of the parent and/or continued vigilance. Even more effective than active techniques are "passive" techniques of injury prevention—techniques that require no active participation on the part of the parent. Examples include requiring safety caps on medicine containers, preventing "right-turn-on-red" in school zones, and raising the local drinking age. Through political advocacy, primary care providers can promote much safer communities for our children. This, too, need not require a great deal of time. Simply offering one's knowledge of accidental injury and accidental injury prevention techniques to concerned civic groups can lead to appropriate legislative initiatives.

Despite the superior effectiveness of "passive" injury prevention methods, active injury prevention strategies should not be overlooked. Active strategies can be divided into those requiring "one-time" action on the part of the parent and those requiring continued vigilance. Examples of the latter would be exercising caution around swimming pools and preventing children from playing with matches. Parallel examples of one-time strategies would be fencing a pool and installing a fire detector. Research has clearly demonstrated the superiority of the one-time injury prevention strategies. Detailed information on injury prevention can be found in the AAP publication entitled *Injury Control*.

Recognition/Access

How does a parent know when an emergency will occur or when a medical condition exists in his or her child that could be a potential emergency? There is no simple answer to this question. Physicians train for years to, among other things, differentiate emergent from nonemergent conditions. It is, nevertheless, easy to forget the perspective of the layperson when it comes to judging the severity of a medical problem. The best answer to the question is that parents must have 24-hour access to medical advice. Preferably this will be provided by the child's primary care physician, either directly or with nursing assistance. In some communities physicians and/or hospitals have spawned "Ask a Nurse" advice lines to fulfill this function. Calling a local emergency department (ED) for advice, however, should be discouraged unless the primary care provider is knowledgeable regarding the quality of the advice provided.

Anticipatory guidance with respect to the recognition of emergency conditions is also important. Once again, however, it is crucial that the layperson's lack of medical sophistication be understood by the advice-giver. Instructions must be simple. Fortunately, the vast majority of emergency conditions in infants and children will manifest themselves in rather marked changes in behavior. Therefore, emphasizing this aspect of a child's condition will greatly assist parents in making proper medical judgments in potential emergency situations. For example, simply instructing a parent to focus on a febrile child's activity level, rather than on the many different associated symptoms such as cough, severity of fever, etc, will generally be the most productive and effective approach to parental recognition of emergency conditions that may be present.

Anticipatory guidance should include advice regarding access to emergency *care*, as well as access to *advice*. In the above scenarios it would be ideal if the primary care providers could rely on the parents to make adequate judgments. Unfortunately, parents may delay with a major injury or medical problem that needs immediate attention. Parents need to know when to access EMS systems. When should a parent proceed to the nearest ED? Which ED is preferred by the primary care physician when there is time to make such a choice? Parents need to be provided with this information. Figure 2 is an example of a handout that can be supplied to parents addressing

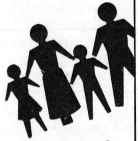

What is a true emergency?

Fortunately, infants and children are not likely to suddenly become seriously ill. Usually there are several early warning signals which will alert you to the need to contact our office for advice before the situation becomes an emergency. If any of the following occur <u>during</u> office hours, immediate notification of our office will allow us to tell you where to go, his/her office or an emergency room. <u>After</u> office hours, notify your doctor and proceed to a hospital emergency room.

- uncontrolled bleeding
- extremely labored breathing
- cyanosis (blue color to the skin or lips)
- convulsions/seizures
- stupor or coma (unconsciousness)
- head injury with transient loss of consciousness or persistent confusion
- fall from a height even without obvious injury
- accidental ingestion of a known poison (Poison Control Center number is: TELEPHONE NUMBER)
- major dental injury (displaced tooth, etc.) obvious broken bone

Provided for your information by:
(NAME AND ADDRESS OF
PHYSICIAN AND/OR HOSPITAL)

Fig 2. Example of handout to guide parents in gaining appropriate access to the EMS system.

For parents of infants, children and adolescents

In Case of
EMERGENCY

─────── **1** ───────

Stay calm. Get help.

─────── **2** ───────

Know the quickest route to both your nearest emergency room and to (NAME OF HOSPITAL).

─────── **3** ───────

If your area is not served by 911, know the number of a nearby ambulance service or county Emergency Medical Service. Inform the Emergency Medical Technicians on the ambulance that you prefer transport to (NAME OF HOSPITAL) if, in their judgment, time permits.

─────── **4** ───────

If you have not already called your physician, instruct the Emergency Department to call your doctor's office or answering service immediately upon your arrival (or instruct someone to call your physician while you are enroute to the hospital). Doctors work closely with Emergency Departments to ensure that the children in our practice receive proper evaluation in an emergency. Also, if another specialist in addition to a Pediatrician is needed, your doctor can be of assistance to the Emergency Department in selecting the most appropriate one for your child.

─────────────

EMERGENCY (TELEPHONE NUMBER)

(NAME OF HOSPITAL AND/OR
PHYSICIAN AND TELEPHONE NUMBER)

these and other questions. Such a handout not only assists parents in gaining appropriate access to the EMS system but also serves to guarantee that the composition of the EMS system chosen by the parent is one that will work both cooperatively and effectively with the child's physician. The cost of producing and printing a handout similar to that illustrated in Figure 2 might reasonably be expected to be shared by the hospital whose ED is recommended in the handout.

As a final note on access, if 911 does not exist in a given community, the primary care providers of that community should be vigorous lobbyists for that service.

First Aid

Anticipatory guidance of parents with respect to emergency care should include some advice regarding emergency first aid. This is best accomplished through simple written material such as the AAP brochure entitled "Choking Prevention and First Aid for Infants and Children." Another example is the publication *Emergency Medical Treatment: Children*, published by the National Safety Council. Verbal instructions are probably most effective when provided as part of a visit for an acute injury or illness. These instructions should be simple and guided by that enduring medical principle: First Do No Harm. For those parents motivated to learn more, the courses produced by the AHA and the American Red Cross, described above, would be excellent sources of information and would include instruction in CPR. Another approach would be to offer locally produced seminars by office personnel for new parents. Appropriate topics would include:

1. Controlling hemorrhage

2. Responding to a choking spell or other respiratory difficulty

3. Helping the child with a seizure

Table 2. — Home First Aid Kit/Cabinet

A lock on the kit or cabinet
Emergency phone number list
Adhesive strips, gauze, adhesive tape, bandage rolls
Antibiotic ointment
Acetaminophen preparations
Syrup of Ipecac
Activated charcoal
Hydrocortisone ointment
Eye patches
Antipruritic (anti-itch) lotion and diphenhydramine
Sling
Elastic bandage
Suction bulb
Thermometer
Splints
Cotton balls, cotton applicators
Hydrogen peroxide
Tweezers, scissors

4. Dealing with a suspected fracture
5. Responding to a severely injured child
6. Managing high fever
7. Caring for minor and moderate burns
8. Evaluating, cleansing, and bandaging a laceration, deep abrasion, or bite wound
9. Caring for eye injuries
10. Ingestions and poisonings

Finally, advice to parents regarding an appropriate home first aid kit would be helpful. Table 2 is an example of a kit that might be recommended to parents; also see Appendix F.

High-Risk Children

Parents of children at high risk for emergency medical conditions, such as the child with a seizure disorder, require a great deal of special education. Other examples of high-risk children include those with asthma, apnea, severe developmental delay, cerebral palsy, sickle cell disease, tracheostomy, and congenital heart disease. All parents of such children should be strongly encouraged to take one of the courses mentioned above. Also, whenever such a patient is hospitalized, one of the goals of the hospitalization should be to educate the parent regarding the prevention, recognition, and immediate first aid of anticipated emergency conditions. The local EMS squad near such a patient's home should also be informed of the potential for an emergency call to that home, the likely emergency medical conditions, and the most appropriate medical treatment. Such children should wear a Medic Alert bracelet. Also, a letter from the primary care provider that is carried by the parent informing emergency caregivers of the child's medical condition and known effective therapies would be helpful. The address of Medic Alert is: Medic Alert Foundation International, PO Box 1009, Turlock, CA 95381-1009; 209/668-3333.

Advocacy

Developing parents into community advocates for an effective EMS system was mentioned previously. Primary care providers, similarly, must use their collective influence to lobby for community policies that promote a safe environment and the resources to respond quickly and effectively when an emergency does occur in a pediatric patient. In particular, with respect to the parent's role, primary care providers need to support community courses on injury prevention and first aid, including CPR, 911, and telephone advice resources.

Action Points

1. Initiate community surveillance of injuries to more effectively provide anticipatory guidance.

2. Encourage all parents to enroll in American Red Cross or AHA-sponsored CPR courses. This is especially important for families with children who have conditions at high risk for respiratory embarrassment.

3. Encourage parents to initiate emergency care should it become necessary.

4. Initiate and sustain anticipatory guidance utilizing all available resources, including the mass media.

5. Provide guidelines for parents regarding when they should contact the office, managed care programs (if appropriate), or 911, and where to seek care (eg, which ED).

6. Provide written instructions to parents regarding appropriate access to the EMS system.

7. Become an advocate for an effective EMS system for children.

AAP Resources

American Academy of Pediatrics, Committee on Accident and Poison Prevention. In: McIntire MS, ed. *Injury Control for Children and Youth.* Elk Grove Village, IL: American Academy of Pediatrics; 1987

American Academy of Pediatrics, Committee on Injury and Poison Prevention: The Injury Prevention Program (TIPP). Elk Grove Village, IL: American Academy of Pediatrics; 1989

American Academy of Pediatrics. *Choking Prevention and First Aid for Infants and Children.* Elk Grove Village, IL: American Academy of Pediatrics; 1990

Bibliography

Agran PF, Dunkle DE, Winn DG. Effects of legislation on motor vehicle injuries to children. *Am J Dis Child.* 1987;141:959-964

Boyce WT, Sprunger LW, Sobolewski S, Schaefer C: Epidemiology of injuries in a large, urban school district. *Pediatrics.* 1984;74:342-349

National Safety Council: *Accident Facts*. Chicago, IL: National Safety Council; 1990

Padilla ER, Rohsenow DJ, Bergman AB. Predicting accident frequency in children. *Pediatrics*. 1976;58:223-226

Rivara FP, Kamitsuka MD, Quan L. Injuries to children younger than 1 year of age. *Pediatrics*. 1988;81:93-97

Runyan CW, Gerken EA. Epidemiology and prevention of adolescent injury: a review and research agenda. *JAMA*. 1989;262:2273-2279

Schaplowsky AF. Community injury control—a management approach. *Am J Public Health*. 1973;63:252-254

Schor EL. Unintentional injuries: patterns within families. *Am J Dis Child*. 1987;141:1280-1284

CHAPTER 4

YOUR OFFICE AS AN EMERGENCY CARE SITE

Case

A 6-month-old infant is brought into your office during the lunch hour with severe wheezing. The mother informs your secretary that she did not believe the infant could wait until her appointment later that afternoon. The infant is retracting; she then becomes cyanotic, begins gasping, and then becomes apneic. What treatment would that child receive in your office if that infant arrived today? What would be the outcome of this infant's emergency?

The previous chapter discussed educating your families about emergency care and emergency services. Your own office staff needs training as well.

Questions

1. Are your nonmedically trained office personnel prepared to respond to this or other emergency situations?
2. Are the medically trained office personnel capable of responding to an emergency within the office setting?

Key Terms

Pediatric Advanced Life Support (PALS): A course was developed conjointly by the American Academy of Pediatrics and the American Heart Association (AHA) with the expressed goal of providing up-to-date information on various aspects of advanced life support for infants and children; the course integrates knowledge and motor skills into a clinically useful discipline.

Advanced Pediatric Life Support (APLS): A course was developed conjointly by the American Academy of

Pediatrics and the American College of Emergency Physicians to provide a core of knowledge in pediatric emergency medicine; the goal of the course is to provide the physician with information necessary to assess and manage critically ill or injured children during the first 30 to 60 minutes in the emergency department (ED). There has been inadequate attention given to the office as an emergency care site. The need for greater emphasis is real. More than 50% of respondents to a 1984 survey at the annual meeting of the Michigan State Medical Society reported multiple occurrences of office events from a defined list of emergencies. The list included emergencies such as anaphylaxis, seizures, insulin reactions, and shock. A similar survey from Chicago investigated pediatrician preparedness. Sixty-two percent of respondents reported that each week they examined more than one child in their offices who required emergency treatment or subsequent hospitalization. Pediatricians in metropolitan Washington, DC, reported treating severe respiratory distress, seizures, obstructed airways, shock, and severe trauma in their offices. Cardiac arrest was uncommon.

It is estimated that fewer than one third of practitioners in a private setting who see urgent cases on a regular basis have adequate equipment and drugs to treat these conditions. The same studies suggest that only 11% of offices are adequately equipped to handle common office emergencies. As an example, one pediatric medical staff survey documented that 25% of offices that administered aerosols or epinephrine for asthma and allergic episodes did not have oxygen availability. A similar percentage of offices that routinely administered parenteral anticonvulsants for active seizures did not have oxygen and bag-and-mask capability. Less than 50% of pediatricians in the Northwest had an office plan for treating emergencies and believed that they were adequately equipped for emergency conditions.

It is our responsibility to ensure that our staffs have the knowledge, training, and resources to respond to office emergencies. This chapter will describe the steps involved in achieving this preparedness.

Triage

Triage is a process of sorting patients according to the urgency of their medical needs. The concept is commonly used in EDs to assign priority to an individual patient.

The office staff must triage patients on the telephone who inquire about illness and must make triage decisions about patients who present for care. The physician must provide leadership and guidance in these matters. If the physician does not set clear expectations, then patients may wait when immediate care is required. It is important that every office have clearly written policies and procedures on telephone management and initial assessment of the patient and a plan detailing appropriate action to take based on this assessment.

It is important that specific guidelines be written by the physician for telephone screening. Every office depends on secretaries, receptionists, and nurses to screen calls during office hours. Many primary care physicians use nurses to screen their calls at night. All persons must be adequately instructed to make an appropriate telephone decision regarding patient disposition. Office personnel should be instructed to determine if a true emergency exists when a call is received. Clear guidelines should exist for actions to be taken depending on whether the physician, a nurse, or only the receptionist is available to answer the call. The receptionist may simply instruct the family to call the Emergency Medical Services (EMS) system. If a nurse or physician is available, the receptionist should have clear instructions to give the call immediately to the available health professional. The nurse could elicit medical information and act according to prescribed algorithms. Commercial telephone triage algorithms have been published and may be used as a reference in establishing your own office protocols. Such protocols are often organized by chief complaint or presenting symptoms. A series of questions allows the triage to assess the severity of the chief complaint and determine the appropriate action. Ready access to the physician for questionable cases is essential. The content of all calls should be documented on a designated form, including recording the specific advice given the family.

Another site for triage is your reception/waiting area. Unfortunately, the first person to assess patients arriving in the office may be the least medically sophisticated employee—your secretary or receptionist. If this is the case, these employees need to be able to recognize emergencies and summon help. Patients who have scheduled appointments may have their conditions deteriorate, as depicted in the case scenario. This can be expected with patients with no scheduled appointments as well. Specific instructions should be given for the situation when no physician is present. For example, can the patient whose condition is deteriorating wait or should EMS be called?

Suggestions for developing a triage program in your practice include:

1. Establish written office policies and procedures for telephone and reception area triage.

2. Ensure that your receptionist determines if an emergency exists before placing a caller on hold.

3. Outline a decision tree for your staff so that true emergencies are referred directly to you, your nurse in your absence, or to the ED, preselected by you.

4. Define those conditions that can be treated in the office and those that should be referred directly to the ED.

5. Provide your staff with instructions on which ED is best suited to deal with these conditions and the names of preferred consultants.

6. Have contingency plans for the staff if no physician is in the office.

7. Train your receptionist to identify infants and children in distress as they register or as their conditions deteriorate in the waiting area.

8. Have the office nurse periodically check the waiting area to assess waiting patients, especially if you are behind schedule.

Preparing Staff

The primary care provider should determine the knowledge and skill level of medical personnel who are newly employed. Nurses, physician's assistants, and other medical providers may have had little exposure to pediatric emergencies in their formal training. It would be unwise to assume that they can recognize the signs and symptoms of serious disease in infants and children or initiate emergency treatment in a time of need.

It is justifiable to expect a quantifiable level of competence in all office care personnel. Enrollment in a CPR course should be mandatory for all office employees. Types and places of enrollment include (1) Basic Life Support course, Module C of the AHA, (2) local hospitals that teach CPR classes for their staffs, and (3) the local AHA or American National Red Cross chapters.

Basic CPR is essential, but medical office personnel should also be able to initiate advanced life support (ALS). Pediatric Advanced Life Support (PALS) courses were introduced by the Academy and the AHA in 1988. This 2-day course emphasizes the recognition and treatment of cardiopulmonary failure, respiratory distress, and shock. Faculty have been appointed in each state in the United States. Local AHA chapters can be contacted for course availability. This course has been well received by physicians, nurses, paramedics, respiratory therapists, and other medical personnel (Appendix G).

The office- or clinic-based physician should supplement such formal training with detailed instructions to the staff with regard to specific pediatric urgencies and emergencies. Recommendations for the emergency treatment of specific situations can be obtained from the growing number of pediatric emergency textbooks and manuals, including the *Advanced Pediatric Life Support Manual* of the Academy. Individual practices can generate their own list of illnesses and treatments. Some suggestions would include respiratory distress—including stridor and wheezing; shock—including dehydration and sepsis; anaphylaxis; seizures; insulin reactions; apnea; and syncope.

Specific protocols should be written in a manual that is readily available. The manual should include step-by-step instructions on actions to be taken, medications needed, and recommended dosages. A specific section explaining the local EMS system should be included. For major emergencies such as anaphylaxis, or apnea, preassigning roles to members of the staff can be invaluable in organizing the resuscitation effort. For example, the office nurse can be responsible for assisting the physician with the airway and giving medications. An aide can be responsible for chest compressions. The secretary can record events and activate the EMS system. Specific models will vary from office to office, depending on expertise, size, and personnel available.

Those personnel who provide telephone communications should receive training in accessing the EMS system. They should be able to provide information needed by the EMS dispatcher. This includes the office's address, patient's age, condition, vital signs (if available), and transport destination. Some jurisdictions have a two-tiered response system—dispatching basic life support (BLS) units prior to advanced life support (ALS) units. The need for an ALS unit should be clearly stated. The same information may be transmitted to the referral ED.

Equipment

Trained personnel need appropriate resources to function effectively. Equipment and medications should be organized so the staff can quickly select the correct equipment and medication based on the child's condition and size. All members of the staff must know the locations of the emergency equipment and supplies.

The physician may choose to organize equipment and medication needs based on height or weight of the child. Equipment and medication should be available to render care for infants and children of all ages. Each office should decide how to stock and resupply the correct materials. Each office should also have a drug dosage chart(s) prominently displayed. The key point is to be organized prior to the development of a crisis situation so that your staff can assist you smoothly in treating emergencies.

Equipping your office for emergencies need not be expensive, as much of the equipment is already available in offices (Table 3). Some offices have a specific procedure or treatment room. In these settings, oxygen and suctioning equipment can be supplied via wall outlets. Alternately, portable oxygen tanks and suction machines can be used. Bag-valve-mask resuscitators or pocket masks with one-way valves should be routinely available to protect the staff from having to perform mouth-to-mouth resuscitation. Reusable bags can be sterilized and appropriate-sized masks stocked. Disposable bag-and-mask sets for use on a single patient are available. Intubation equipment is optional, depending on the office setting and comfort level of the physician.

Circulatory support equipment is relatively inexpensive. Catheters requiring guidewires can be placed in the external jugular or femoral vein, if the physician is trained in this technique. Rapid vascular access can often be obtained using standard intravenous (IV) catheters or an intraosseous needle. The monitoring equipment listed as

Table 3. — Suggested Supply and Equipment List

Airway Management
- Oxygen source with flowmeter
- Oxygen masks—preemie, infant, child, adult
- Bag-valve-mask resuscitators, including reservoir—infant, child, adult
- Suction—wall or machine
- Suction catheters—Yankauer, 8, 10, 14F
- Oral airways—0-5
- Nasal cannulas—infant, child, and adult sizes 1-3
- Optional for intubation
    - Laryngoscope handle with Miller blades—0, 1, 2, 3
    - Endotracheal tubes, uncuffed—3.0, 3.5, 4.0, 4.5, 5.0, 6.0, 7.0, 8.0
    - Stylets—small, large
    - Magill forceps

Fluid Management
- Intraosseous needles—15- and 18-gauge
- IV catheters, short, over the needle—20-, 22-, 24-gauge
- Butterfly needles—21-, 23-, 25-gauge
- IV boards, tape, alcohol swabs, tourniquet
- Pediatric drip chambers and tubing
- D5 one-half normal saline
- Isotonic fluids (normal saline or lactated Ringer's solution)
- Optional: over guidewire catheters 3, 4, 5F

Miscellaneous Equipment
- Blood pressure cuffs—preemie infant, child, adult
- Nasogastric tubes—10, 14F
- Feeding tubes—3, 5F
- Foley catheters—8, 10F
- Sphygmomanometer
- Cardiac arrest board

Optional Equipment
- Portable monitor defibrillator
- Doppler
- Noninvasive blood pressure monitor
- Pulse oximeter

Table 4. — Suggested Medications for Treating Emergencies in the Office

Aqueous adrenalin—1:1000, 1:10,000
Dextrose in water—25%, 50%
Atropine sulfate
Sodium bicarbonate—4.2%, 8.4%
Calcium chloride—10%
Lorazepam or diazepam
Phenobarbital
Antibiotics, parenteral
Diphenhydramine, parenteral
Methylprednisolone
Naloxone
Ipecac
Activated charcoal
Albuterol for inhalation
L-epinephrine for nebulizer

optional is expensive and should not be necessary in most office settings.

Medications should be available to treat allergic, respiratory, and circulatory emergencies. Seizures and ingestions are also common (Table 4). Medications and supplies should be routinely inspected for expiration dates and supply levels. There should be a card documenting that emergency supplies have been checked on a weekly or biweekly basis. Restocking should be performed after each emergency.

Physician Skills

The physician must be comfortable with airway management and circulatory support. The office practitioner cares for true emergencies on an infrequent basis. Maintaining skills requires practice and commitment. Fortunately, there are an increasing number of CME opportunities in pediatric emergencies. Many institutions offer "first 30-minute" courses in the stabilization and transport of infants and children. The previously mentioned Pediatric Advanced Life Support (PALS) course teaches resuscitation. The Advanced Pediatric Life Support course (APLS) of the Academy/American College of Emergency Physicians includes a textbook, laboratory, and small group sessions devoted to common urgent and emergent pediatric conditions.

Some physicians maintain skills by "moonlighting" or working part-time in an area ED, often alongside a staff emergency physician or pediatric emergency physician. An excellent method of staying current is to become a PALS or APLS instructor. Some medical centers provide short-term preceptorships for practicing physicians. Other worthwhile courses include Advanced Cardiac Life Support sponsored by the AHA and Advanced Trauma Life Support sponsored by the American College of Surgeons. Thus, there are an increasing number of options for the physician who is concerned about maintaining resuscitative abilities.

Keeping Prepared

Maintaining a state of readiness is a difficult task. The initial enthusiasm generated by courses wanes with time, as does retention of skills and knowledge. Periodic update becomes important. This may involve refresher courses. Most nationally recognized certifications are for 2 years, with a requirement for an update course.

Basic CPR certification is renewable every 2 years, but it is advisable to require annual recertification of your staff. "Mock codes" are commonly used in hospitals to maintain and reinforce readiness. This could easily be done in the office setting as well. The physician creates a scenario such as the case presented in which a child has respiratory failure. Staff members respond to their assigned tasks while the physician directs events. Team members then critique their performances. Specific action plans for improvement and problem solving should result from such an effort. Scavenger hunts are also useful. A staff member is given a list of items needed in an emergency and given a set time, eg, 5 minutes, to find them. This helps assure that your staff will be able to respond quickly in an emergency. Often problems in stocking or ordering are uncovered in this manner. Suggestions for your preparation include:

1. Properly organize and maintain emergency equipment and supplies.

2. Prepare a resuscitation equipment/medication system based on patient's weight or height.

3. Take a pediatric emergencies course, eg, APLS.

4. Become a PALS or APLS instructor.

5. Work occasional shifts in an ED.

6. Enroll in an Advanced Cardiac Life Support or Advanced Trauma Life Support course.

7. Require periodic recertification of your staff.

8. Practice mock resuscitations with your staff.

9. Send your staff on scavenger hunts.

10. Maintain a basic library of pediatric emergency medicine references (Appendix H).

Documentation of Emergency Care

Careful, complete, and accurate documentation of your emergency care is important for ongoing patient care and may be vital if you become entangled with the legal system or disciplinary boards. Major malpractice judgments have been handed down due to poor record keeping. Physicians have had their licenses suspended due to a failure to resuscitate patients properly. Yet emergency situations are the most difficult to document properly. Stress levels are high. There are often not enough trained assistants. When the crisis passes, the angry, tired, and disgruntled patients who fill the waiting room remain to be treated and soothed. Writing or dictating a record seems low in priority.

It is important to take the time immediately following the emergency to document the events. The sequence of actions are still fresh in your mind. Charting done days to weeks later may not be as accurate. A recorder during the event can be invaluable. Most hospital resuscitation teams have a nurse assigned solely to that task. Perhaps an aide or secretary could write orders given and note times, allowing you to better reconstruct the timing and sequence of your interventions. Another helpful method, if available, is to turn on your pocket dictaphone. Verbal orders and treatments will be recorded, allowing you to reconstruct events accurately.

Written records are acceptable but must be legible. Dictated and typed notes are usually more complete and legible. The notes should record the date and time written or dictated as well as the time of the event. A complete record should be made of the history, physical examination, and any treatment given. Commenting on the rationale for treatment and the diagnoses considered can be helpful in the future. Consultations obtained by telephone or in person should be noted. It is important to record stabilization attempts and requests for transfer and transport. The timing of these phone calls may become important if there is a delay in ambulance availability or refusal by an institution to accept the patient in transfer. Record any conversations or explanations given the family. Document the patient's condition at the time of departure from your office. This documentation could be vital to you if an adverse outcome occurs.

Documentation of the steps you have taken to keep yourself and your staff trained and ready can also be important. Keep records of courses attended and your own lectures to the staff in each employee's personnel file. Record the dates and attendance at drills and scavenger hunts. Have written personnel policies requiring necessary certifications. These efforts will help in dealing with the legal system and also in organizing your office's approach to emergency care.

Suggestions for documentation include:

1. Designate a recorder during the resuscitation, if possible. Alternately, record the resuscitation effort.

2. Write or dictate your notes as soon as possible, preferably immediately after the event.

3. Record dates and times of treatments, calls for transport, and transfer.

4. Document the patient's condition at the time of leaving your care.

5. Document your program for office preparedness.

Action Points

1. Develop a telephone triage protocol for all persons who answer the office telephone.

2. Train office personnel to identify children who are acutely injured or ill.

3. Develop protocols for treatment of specific emergencies that may be encountered in the office. Include methods for accurate calculation of drug doses based on height or weight. The Pediatric Resuscitation Measuring Tape developed by James Broselow, MD, can be used to determine drug dosages and equipment needs for pediatric patients. Different color zones on one side of the tape indicate recommended equipment sizes. On the other side of the tape recommended drug dosages are shown by Kilograms that correspond to the normal weight at that length (Appendix I).*

---

*These tapes can be ordered by contacting Armstrong Medical Industries, Inc, at 575 Knightsbridge Parkway, PO Box 700, Lincolnshire, IL 60069-0700; 800/323-4220 or 708/913-0101.

4. Assure basic life support training for the entire office staff.

5. Provide current advanced life support training for office personnel who provide assistance with patient care.

6. Write protocols for accessing the EMS system.

7. Secure and maintain a full complement of emergency equipment within the office.

8. Practice mock drills with your office staff.

AAP Resources

Silverman BK, ed. *Advanced Pediatric Life Support*. Elk Grove Village, IL: American Academy of Pediatrics; Dallas, TX: American College of Emergency Physicians; 1989

Chameides L, ed. *Textbook of Pediatric Advanced Life Support*. Dallas, TX: American Heart Association; 1988

Bibliography

Altieri M, Bellet J, Scott H. Preparedness for pediatric emergencies encountered in the practitioner's office. *Pediatrics*. 1990;85:710-714

Baker MD, Ludwig S. Pediatric emergency transport and the private practitioner. *Pediatrics*. 1991;88:691-695

Fuchs S, Jaffe DM, Christoffel KK. Pediatric emergencies in office practices: prevalence and office preparedness. *Pediatrics*. 1989;83:931-939

Hodge D III. Pediatric emergency office equipment. *Pediatr Emerg Care*. 1988;4:212-214

Katz HP. Medical care by telephone. In: Dershewitz RA. *Ambulatory Pediatric Care*. Philadelphia, PA: JB Lippincott Co; 1988:18-23

Lubitz DS, Seidel JS, Chameides L, Luten RC, Zaritsky AL, Campbell FW. A rapid method for estimating weight and resuscitation drug dosages from length in the pediatric age group. *Ann Emerg Med*. 1988;17:576-581

Schweich PJ, DeAngelis C, Duggan AK. Preparedness of practicing pediatricians to manage emergencies. *Pediatrics*. 1991;88:223-229

CHAPTER 5

PREHOSPITAL TRANSPORT OF YOUR PATIENT

Cases

A 4-year-old runs out into the street and is hit by a car in a quiet suburban town somewhere in America. A bystander calls 911 and moments later an ambulance arrives. Out steps a young basic emergency medical technician in uniform.

An 18-month-old, temporarily unwatched, falls into a swimming pool in southern California. The infant is pulled from the swimming pool and is not breathing. A neighbor starts CPR and 911 is called. An ambulance with a paramedic arrives moments later.

Questions

1. Which responder has the capacity to evaluate, treat, and transport these pediatric patients?
2. Will both of these prehospital care providers be able to appropriately provide stabilizing care and transport these children?
3. How can the primary care provider influence the care administered by these prehospital care workers?

Key Terms

Basic Emergency Medical Technician (EMT): A prehospital care provider who has a total of 100 to 120 hours of education, of which 10 hours (on the average) are devoted to pediatric clinical and didactic instruction.

Emergency Medical Technician-Paramedic (EMT-P): A paramedic, a care provider who has had 1,000 or more hours of instruction.

This chapter describes the various personnel who deliver, possibly vital, care before a child is brought to the hospital and describes their role in providing emergency medical services for children.

Prehospital care may be delivered to acutely ill or injured children by parents, first responders, fire or police personnel, EMTs, paramedics, and any combination of the above. Even those trained to handle emergencies are often lacking in specific training or experience to care for children. All who may find themselves tending to a critically ill child should have some training to address children's special needs.

Personnel

First responders who are either volunteers or paid employees such as police officers, firefighters, or other public servants should have training in first aid and CPR. Their purpose is to provide basic intervention until more skilled and better equipped personnel arrive. Their knowledge base may be restricted to a basic CPR course, or be as extensive as a 40- to 60-hour course of instruction. The official first-responder course developed by the National Highway Traffic Safety Administration requires 40 hours of training. In all these courses, the pediatric portion of the programs received insufficient emphasis. Primary care providers would do well to promote the completion of separate CPR courses concentrating on infant CPR and prevention strategies for these first responders.

Most ambulances in this country are staffed by basic EMTs or first responders. These highly motivated laypersons seek training, certification, and ongoing medical education, and take calls, all out of a sense of civic duty. The same cadre of persons are often the volunteer firefighters of their areas. Many urban and heavily populated suburban areas run professional ambulance services using full-time career EMTs. Many of these persons will, in addition, work as volunteer EMTs in their communities. The level of training of these persons varies widely. To become a certified emergency medical technician-ambulance (EMT-A) requires 100 hours of training; this training allows the person to evaluate the patient's ABCs, mental status, and general level of distress. The EMT is trained to deliver oxygen; perform bag-valve-mask ventilation, CPR, spinal immobilization; handle splint fractures; and apply military antishock trousers. Recently, there has been a move toward supplying basic EMT-As with training to use an automatic defibrillator. Such training provides a certification of EMT-D.

Higher levels of EMTs are trained to deliver more advanced medical intervention in the prehospital setting. Ranging from EMT-2 to the highest level, the paramedic (EMT-P), these paraprofessionals are trained to perform tasks, under medical control, previously considered to be only in the domain of the physician. The tasks vary by locale, but paramedics are trained to intubate, establish vascular access using intravenous and intraosseous infusion needles, deliver medications, defibrillate, deliver nebulized medication, place nasogastric tubes and, in some systems, perform needle thoracotomy and needle cricothyroidotomy. Despite the availability of advanced training, in many systems children are excluded from receiving advanced life support. Also, in some locales, children are treated under the same protocols written for adults. Ambulance dispatchers have variable training. They may be EMTs, paramedics, or registered nurses. Any given system in a community or region may be only basic life support (BLS) capable, or advanced life support (ALS) and BLS capable (a two-tiered system). Few communities have only ALS services. The dispatcher who functions in a two-tiered system has the task of assigning a call either to an ALS or BLS unit, depending on the nature of the call, in other words, to perform telephone triage. This type of triage is usually guided by written protocols. It is increasingly common for these operators to offer telephone medical guidance to families awaiting the arrival of an ambulance.

It has been documented that most EMTs, paramedics in the field, as well as ambulance dispatchers have inadequate training in the special needs of children in the prehospital setting. Many responders in parts of the country lack equipment to deliver BLS or ALS to children. These deficiencies are now being addressed in many regions of this country; however, most communities are not yet benefiting from improved pediatric training to those providing prehospital care.

Triage

In an ideal system, each child would be appropriately triaged in the field and brought to the proper medical facility by an appropriately trained prehospital provider. Unfortunately, this does not describe reality even in the most developed of systems. Even in locales with excellent prehospital systems, large numbers of children continue to be transported by parents, neighbors, police officers, and untrained providers, perhaps to facilities without the necessary expertise or equipment to stabilize a critically ill or injured child.

Medical Control

A key aspect to improve care for children by prehospital personnel is to provide input into medical control both directly and indirectly (see Chapter 2). In the majority of systems there is a physician committee that provides input and collaborates on writing and modifying treatment protocols, triage criteria, and equipment lists. This form of indirect medical control exists even when the system has a medical director. This is an excellent forum for the primary care provider to become involved with in order to advocate for the special needs of children. Of interest is the lack of pediatric input at this level that occurred during the initial development of EMS, which resulted in an adult-oriented system that did not recognize children's needs.

Although a few systems provide pediatric direct medical control, the vast majority do not have the capability to do so. Therefore, the physicians providing the direct medical control require training and exposure to pediatric emergency medicine to provide appropriate guidance to ambulance dispatchers, EMTs, and paramedics caring for children.

Equipment

A national survey performed by Seidel et al revealed a tremendous variability in pediatric equipment inventory carried by EMS agencies throughout the United States. The majority were clearly deficient. Tables 5-7 adapted from the American College of Emergency Physicians, suggest minimum requirements to equip for BLS and ALS care. Certainly more sophisticated systems might see fit to include items for monitoring (ie, pulse oximeter) and/or pain control (nitrous oxide delivery system). In the majority of cases, the primary care provider will want to assure that appropriate, minimum equipment is available and training for its use adequate.

Action Points

Primary care providers should improve EMS by:

1. Advocating additional training specific to pediatrics for those responders who have less than 100 hours of training.
2. Assuring that the responders in their community and region have appropriate equipment.
3. Directly offering their services for both indirect and direct medical control. As an alternative, they may wish to provide guidance to medical committees that implement and modify patient protocols.
4. Checking the infant and children equipment inventories for their local squads.

Table 5. — Basic Life Support: Minimum Pediatric Equipment and Supplies

Equipment

- Oxygen tank with tubing, with humidified source for long transport times
- Oral airways—sizes 0-5F
- Nasopharyngeal airways with lubricant—12F-30F or equivalent sizes in millimeters
- Self-inflating bags with oxygen reservoir—250-, 500-, or 1000-ml bags
- Oxygen reservoir masks—infant, child, adult
- Nasal cannulas—infant, child, adult sizes 1-3
- Masks for bag-valve-mask—infant, child, adult sizes 1-3
- Stethoscope
- Blood pressure cuffs—infant, child, adult
- Portable suction unit
- Suction catheters (flexible and rigid)—6F-14F
- Back board for spinal immobilization—short and long board
- Equipment for neck immobilization
- Towel rolls/blanket rolls/or equivalent
- Rigid cervical collar (for children more than 2 y —infant, child, small, medium, adult)
- Femur splint—designed for pediatric patients
- Burn pack—standard pack; towels or gel burn sheet acceptable
- Thermal absorbent blanket
- Equipment sizing tape or equipment/age/weight chart
- Heat source for ambulance compartment

Supplies

- Adhesive tape
- Alcohol sponges
- Arm boards—various sizes
- Providine-iodine preparation pads
- Elastic bandages
- Extra batteries and bulbs for equipment needs
- Flashlight, bulb, batteries
- Gauze rolls
- Gauze sponges
- Protective eyewear, gloves, masks
- Scissors
- Tincture of benzoin
- Tongue blades

Table 6. — Advanced Life Support: Minimum Pediatric Equipment and Medications

BLS minimum equipment and supplies, plus following equipment

Monitoring

> Transport monitor—battery-operated with 3 or 4 lead wires
> Defibrillator with 4.25- and 8-cm paddles (or paddle adapter) and pads capable to dial down to appropriate watt-sec for pediatric patients. When replacing current equipment, new equipment should have settings below 25 watt-sec.
> Monitoring electrodes
> Equipment and drug dosage tape or age-weight chart
> Glucose detection strips

Airway

> Laryngoscope handle with extra batteries and bulbs
> Laryngoscope blades—straight and/or curved, 0, 1, 2, 3
> Stylettes—pediatric sizes
> Endotracheal tubes
> Uncuffed ranges 3.0-5.5
> Cuffed range 5.0-8.0
> Magill forceps (Rachevsky)
> Lubrication (water soluble)
> Nasogastric tube—sizes 5F-18F

Vascular Access

> Intravenous catheter of choice—16-22 gauge
> Intraosseous needles of choice
> Tourniquet/rubber bands
> 3-way stopcocks or adapter that allows administration of additional fluids or medications
> Syringes—various sizes
> Blood sample tubes
> Intravenous tubing, microdrop delivery system
> Tuberculin syringes

Intravenous Solutions

> Normal saline or lactated Ringer's
> D5W (diluent)
> Sodium chloride—bacteriostatic, for injection
> Water—bacteriostatic, for injection

Table 6. — Advanced Life Support: Minimum Pediatric Equipment and Medications (continued)

Medications/Concentrations
> Atropine sulfate—0.1 mg/mL
> Bicarbonate, sodium—8.4% (1.0 mEq/mL)
> Diazepam or analeptic of choice—5 mg/mL
> Epinephrine—1:1000 (1 mg/mL)
> Epinephrine—1:10,000 (0.1 mg/mL)
> Lidocaine hydrochloride (IV)—10 mg/mL
> Naloxone hydrochloride (adult)—1.0 mg/mL
> Pain medication per medical control
> D50 (dextrose 50 + water and diluent)
> Inhalant beta-adrenergic agent of choice
> Activated charcoal
> Drug dose chart based on length, age, or weight

Table 7. — Basic and Advanced Life Support Minimum Resuscitation Equipment and Supplies for the Newborn

Basic Life Support for Newborn
> Oxygen cylinder
> Stethoscope
> Bulb syringe
> Portable suction
> Suction catheters—5F-10F range
> Resuscitation bag— 750 mL (250 mL or 500 mL)
> Face mask (infant)—premature and newborn sizes
> Gauze
> Sterile scissors
> Thermal absorbent blanket and head cover
> Cord clamps
> Appropriate heat source for ambulance compartment

Advance Life Support for Newborn
> BLS equipment for newborn as listed above, plus:
> Endotracheal tube uncuffed—3.0-4.0 mm
> Endotracheal tube stylet—6F
> Laryngoscope—straight blades 0 and 1
> Infusion set, microdrip unit

AAP Resources

Luten R, Foltin G, eds. *Pediatric Resources for Prehospital Care*. Elk Grove Village, IL: American Academy of Pediatrics; 1990

Bibliography

Barkin RM. Pediatrics in the emergency medical services system. *Pediatr Emerg Care*. 1990;6:72-77

Haller JA, ed. *Emergency Medical Services for Children: Report of the 97th Ross Conference on Pediatric Research*. Columbus, OH: Ross Laboratories. 1989:1-145

National Highway Traffic Safety Administration. *Emergency Medical Services: 1990 and Beyond*. Washington, DC: NHTSA; October 1990. US Dept of Transportation Publication DOT HS 807-639

Seidel JS. Emergency medical services and the pediatric patient: are the needs being met? II: training and equipping emergency medical services providers for pediatric emergencies. *Pediatrics*. 1986;78:808-812

Seidel JS, Hornbein M, Yoshiyama K, Kuznets D, Finklestein JZ, St Geme JW, Jr. Emergency medical services and the pediatric patient: are the needs being met? *Pediatrics*. 1984;73:769-772

CHAPTER 6

COMMUNITY HOSPITAL EMERGENCY DEPARTMENTS

Cases

A 26-month-old girl is found unresponsive after submersion in a swimming pool for an unknown period of time and is brought to the community hospital emergency department (ED). She has no primary care physician and you are on call for the ED panel this Saturday afternoon.

A 7-year-old boy that you have known since birth falls off of a cliff, is unresponsive, has a Glasgow Coma Score of 9, and is brought to the community hospital ED by paramedics.

A mother of a 5-year-old patient of yours who has a seizure disorder calls the office and tells the nurse that her son is in the ED of a hospital across town and has had seizures for 45 minutes.

A 10-year-old boy falls off of his bicycle and is brought to the ED by a neighbor who calls to say he has a fractured femur.

Questions

1. Are the EDs in your community hospitals staffed and equipped to offer optimum emergency care and critical care to all of the patients in the scenarios presented above?
2. What are the resources that community hospitals should have in place to manage pediatric emergencies?
3. What is the role of the pediatric community in assuring that the special needs of infants, children, and adolescents are met by the hospitals that are used for pediatric care?

This chapter will answer these and other questions about the community hospital as a component of the emergency medical services (EMS) system.

Key Terms

Emergency Department Approved for Pediatrics (EDAP): Defines a facility with an institutional and professional staff commitment to provide care for the ill or injured child.

Local Pediatric Center (LPC): A hospital with secondary or tertiary pediatric care capabilities.

Pediatric Critical Care Center (PCC): A hospital with the complete spectrum of pediatric subspecialty services, including pediatric trauma.

About 10% of the prehospital care calls are made for patients in the pediatric age group and the majority of these patients are transported to community hospital EDs by the EMS system. Most EMS protocols dictate that emergency medical technicians and paramedics transport patients to the "nearest appropriate facility." In some systems specific pediatric critical care centers, specialty centers (eg, pediatric trauma centers), and pediatric EDs have been identified by the regional or local EMS agency, and these facilities are used whenever possible for pediatric emergency care. In many states, regions, and local areas, there is no definition as to what constitutes a "pediatric patient," which may add confusion to the designation protocols for EMS provider agencies.

The majority of infants, children, and adolescents are brought to the ED by their caretakers: parents, relatives, or foster parents. A small number come to the ED accompanied by school nurses, babysitters, social workers, or law enforcement personnel, which may present a special problem with consent for care (see Chapter 9, "Planning for Special Situations").

The Organization of the Community Emergency Department

Pediatric patients who make a self-referral with and without a caretaker or who are brought in for care via an EMS provider must be triaged by an experienced nurse or physician. Clerical personnel are not trained to determine illness or injury acuity and should not be put in this position. The patient's chief complaint, general appearance, and behavior, particularly as it pertains to the caretaker and the environment, should be assessed along with vital signs. Weight and height should also be taken. *No patients should be dismissed or referred for evaluation elsewhere without first being assessed by a health care professional.*

After the patient is triaged and the level of care needed determined to be emergency, urgent, or nonurgent, the child may be placed in a monitored bed, in a pediatric treatment area, or sent to the waiting area. For instance, the patients with status epilepticus, near drowning, and multiple trauma are emergencies and should be taken to a monitored bed with concurrent evaluation and treatment. The child with an isolated femur fracture should be taken to the pediatric treatment area. Patients who are deemed less critical can safely stay in the waiting area, which ideally is visible from the nursing station.

In many instances pediatric patients receiving care in EDs have a primary care provider or belong to managed care programs. The physicians and nurses in the ED may not be aware of this health care professional unless the registration procedure specifically asks for that information or the caretaker offers it to the treating health care persons. It is thus important that the collection of this information be part of the ED protocol. The primary physician may wish to be part of the treating team or may have valuable information about the health status of a particular child. For instance, the 5-year-old patient in status epilepticus described above may only respond to certain medications. The 7-year-old child with multiple injuries may have asthma, which may complicate the airway management. The primary care provider should also be used for follow-up care for children seen in the ED.

Pediatricians and pediatric subspecialists should be on all community hospital ED call panels. Complicated problems often require consultation with a general pediatrician or pediatric medical or surgical subspecialist. In many rural and remote communities pediatric consultation is not immediately available. However, most pediatric centers generally provide consultative services through their EDs or pediatric intensive care units.

We must remember that emergency medicine is a relatively new specialty and pediatric emergency medicine a very new subspecialty. Thus we cannot expect that all hospitals will have physicians experienced in the assessment of pediatric emergencies on duty at all times. Additionally, not all acute care community hospitals in the country have their EDs staffed with physicians and nurses who have specialized training in emergency medicine. Even physicians who are board-prepared or board-certified in emergency medicine may not have been exposed to an extensive curriculum in pediatric emergency medicine.

Irrespective of physician training, a readily available pediatric reference library may prove beneficial and is suggested for all facilities that render pediatric care (Appendix H).

The care of pediatric patients requires additional assessment skills and it is important that the nursing and physician staff have these skills. If the 7-year-old who fell and was brought to the ED unconscious experienced respiratory distress, it would be important that the ED staff could assess the etiology—neurologic injury, a metabolic problem, or his asthma. A survey of the nursing staffs of 30 rural hospitals in northern California demonstrated that nurses were least comfortable with their knowledge and skills in caring for children under 5 years of age, especially those with respiratory problems.

Emergency departments must also have equipment and supplies that are appropriate to the care of infants, children, and adolescents (Table 8). These include equipment for assessment, such as a pediatric scale, blood pressure cuffs of appropriate size, and various sizes of oxygen masks, laryngoscope blades, and endotracheal tubes. If the 7-year-old in the case scenario needs endotracheal intubation, the appropriate equipment and supplies must be immediately available. The supplies must be organized so that age-appropriate equipment and supplies are immediately available. The system for organizing the supplies may be by weight or using the Broselow tape (Appendix I), which relies on a relationship between height and weight.

The hospital environment is very important in alleviating children's fears. Children respond to familiar surroundings such as pictures of heroes, Ninja Turtles, etc. Optimally, ED design should take into consideration the special needs of children when planning the patient care environment. A separate pediatric room or designated bed can be decorated appropriately. The area should be large enough to allow the caretaker to stay with the child. It should also be in view of the nursing station so that continuous monitoring and assessment is possible. Children should be shielded from viewing potentially psychologically traumatic situations.

Protocols, policies, and procedures for the care of children in the ED are also necessary. An example of standards and guidelines for a general community hospital that are modified from the Los Angeles County Project for setting standards for emergency departments approved for pediatrics/pediatric critical care (EDAP/PCC) are shown (Table 8). The development of these standards was originally a joint project of the Los Angeles Pediatric Society, California Chapter 2 of the American Academy of Pediatrics, and the

Table 8. — Standards for Emergency Departments Approved for Pediatrics (EDAP)*

Definition: An Emergency Department Approved for Pediatrics (EDAP) is a licensed basic emergency department (physician on duty 24 hours) that meets specific minimum standards in order to provide emergency pediatric care. The specific professional staff and equipment standards are as follows.

Professional Staff: Physicians

Standard Requirements

1.1 All physicians who are not board-certified or board-prepared[†] in Emergency Medicine shall have successfully completed the AHA Advanced Cardiac Life Support (ACLS) course as specified by the Joint Commission on Accreditation of Healthcare Organizations. New hospital employees shall complete the ACLS provider course within a reasonable time, not to exceed 3 months from date of employment. This requirement may be met by completion of the AHA Pediatric Advanced Life Support course or the AAP-ACEP Advanced Pediatric Life Support (APLS) course.

1.2 All full-time[‡] emergency physicians and pediatricians who are not board-certified or board-prepared[†] in their respective fields must have documentation of completion of 4 hours of CME in pediatric topics annually. CME shall be accumulated for the first year of this requirement by June 1, 1989. This requirement may be fulfilled by the AHA PALS course or by the AAP-ACEP APLS course. It is recommended that all physicians regularly assigned to the ED fulfill a CME requirement of 4 hours of pediatric topics per year.

1.3 At least 75% of the ED coverage shall be provided by physicians (including senior residents) functioning as emergency physicians on a full-time basis (minimum 96 hours per month in an ED) or by pediatricians experienced in emergency care. Residents "moonlighting" outside of their assigned facility do not meet this requirement.

1.4 At least 50% of the ED coverage shall be provided by physicians (1) board-certified in either emergency medicine or pediatrics, or (2) qualified to sit for the certifying exam in emergency medicine, or (3) who have completed the written examination and are actively pursuing certification in pediatrics.

1.5 One member of a panel of pediatricians, who is board-certified in pediatrics, or who has completed the written examination and is actively pursuing certification in pediatrics, shall be on call 24 hours/day to the EDAP.

1.6 At least one additional emergency physician shall be on call and available within 30 minutes to assist in critical situations.

1.7 A designated Pediatric Quality Assurance Consultant, (1) board-certified in pediatrics, or (2) who has completed the written examination and is actively pursuing certification in pediatrics, shall be available to the EDAP. The Pediatric Quality Assurance Consultant is responsible for participating with the ED physician in quality assurance activities. Quality assurance review shall include all ED pediatric deaths and all pediatric full arrests and be supported by appropriate documentation.

1.8 A representative of the Department of Pediatrics shall sit on the Emergency Care Committee of the hospital. If the hospital does not have a Department of Pediatrics, this requirement may be met by the Pediatric Quality Assurance Consultant sitting on the Committee.

1.9 An on-call panel of physicians available for immediate consultation to the ED to include: anesthesia, pediatric surgery, orthopedics, urology, neurosurgery, pediatric neurology, ophthalmology, head and neck surgery, radiology.

Professional Staff: Nursing

Standard Requirements

2.1 At least 1 registered nurse (RN) per shift shall have successfully completed the AHA PALS or ACLS Provider course. New hospital employees shall complete the PALS or ACLS provider training program within a reasonable time, not to exceed 3 months from date of employment. This requirement may be met by successful completion of the AAP-ACEP APLS course.

2.2 A Pediatric Liaison Nurse (PdLN) shall be designated. This nurse may be shared between institutions and may be employed in other areas of the hospital such as ward, ICU, nursery, or quality assurance. This nurse shall have at least 2 years' experience in pediatrics and/or quality assurance. Responsibilities of the PdLN include:

2.2.1 Ensuring and documenting ED nurse pediatric continuing education (see Standard 2.4).

2.2.2 Maintaining a log and coordinating criteria-based review and follow-up of a sample of pediatric emergency visits. This sample shall include all pediatric full arrests, all pediatric ED deaths, and all pediatric emergencies transported by the paramedics.

2.2.3 Completion of 8 hours of continuing education units (CEU) approved by the Board of Registered Nursing (BRN) in pediatric topics per year. The CEUs shall be accumulated for the first year of this requirement by September 1988.

2.2.4 Coordination of the review of paramedic-transported pediatric cases with the Paramedic Liaison Nurse in hospitals where the EDAP is also the paramedic base station, including tape reviews of pediatric runs.

Table 8. — Standards for Emergency Departments Approved for Pediatrics (EDAP)* (continued)

2.3 At least 1 RN per shift shall have completed a postgraduate course in pediatrics or shall have at least 1 year's experience as an RN caring for pediatric patients in a pediatric emergency department, pediatric ward, or pediatric intensive care unit. It is recommended that *all* ED nurses meet this requirement.

2.4 All nurses regularly assigned to the ED shall attend a minimum of 4 hours BRN-approved pediatric topics per year.

Policies and Procedures

Standard Requirements

3.1 Policies and procedures concerning the transfer of critically ill and injured patients to Pediatric Critical Care Centers or other specialty centers; Level 2 and 3 neonatal, burn, replantation, and behavioral emergencies.

3.2 Policies and procedures for the identification, evaluation, and referral of victims of suspected child abuse.

3.3 Policies and procedures for death of a child and Sudden Infant Death Syndrome.

3.4 Policies and procedures for organ donation.

3.5 Policies and procedures for immunosuppressed patients presenting to the ED for care.

3.6 Policies and procedures for reporting infectious diseases on the County Confidential Morbidity Report Cards.

Equipment, trays, and supplies

Standard Requirements for Equipment

4.1 Pediatric bag-valve resuscitation device

4.2 Transparent masks to use with bag-valve device in preemie, infant, child, and adult sizes

4.3 Laryngoscope with infant and child laryngoscope blades, curved and straight (sizes 0-3)

4.4 Pediatric Magill forceps

4.5 Cervical spine immobilization devices (sand bags, stiff neck headbed, etc). Rigid four-post or plastic/Velcro collars in sizes for children and adults

4.6 Pediatric femur splint (pediatric antishock garments may be used to fulfill this requirement)

4.7 Blood warmer

4.8 An infant warming procedure/device

4.9 Infusion pumps, drip, or volumetric

4.10 Pediatric bone marrow needles for intraosseous infusion

4.11 Blood pressure cuffs: infant, child, adult, and thigh sizes

4.12 Doppler-sensing device for blood pressure measurement

4.13 Monitor-defibrillator with 0-400 W/s capability

4.14 Pediatric scale

4.15 An appropriate procedure/device for ensuring pediatric restraint

Standard Requirements for Trays

4.16 Pediatric thoracotomy tray, including pediatric rib-spreader and aortic clamp

4.17 Pediatric tracheostomy tray with tracheostomy tubes (sizes 0-3)

4.18 Setup for needle cricothyrotomy (3.5 Portex adapter and 14-gauge over-the-needle catheter acceptable)

4.19 Venesection tray appropriate for infants and children

4.20 Peritoneal lavage tray

4.21 Pediatric lumbar puncture trays with 22-gauge, 1.5-in spinal needle

Standard Requirements for Supplies

4.22 Pediatric oral airways (sizes 0-5)

4.23 Endotracheal tubes (sizes 2.5-9.0)

4.24 Chest tubes sizes (16-28F; size 26 unavailable)

4.25 Pediatric suction catheters (sizes 6-12F)

4.26 Central venous catheters (22-14 gauge)

4.27 Pediatric IV supplies, including volumetric sets, butterflies, and over-the-needle catheters: 25-gauge through 14-gauge; 250 mL or 500 mL bags of NS, D5/0.25 NS, D5/0.5 NS, D5 NS, D10/W

4.28 Printed pediatric drug dosage reference material (calculated on dose-per-kilogram basis), readily available, preferably on a wall-mounted chart or the Broselow tape system of drug dosing by length

4.29 Sodium bicarbonate, in 10 mEq/10 mL pre-filled syringes

4.30 All drugs currently recommended for pediatric and adult resuscitation by the AHA

4.31 Pediatric nasogastric tubes, including sizes 3.0-and 5.0-F infant feeding tubes

4.32 Pediatric Foley catheters (size 8-22F)

Quality Assurance and Data Collection

Standard Requirements

5.1 A written quality assurance plan with a pediatric component that includes the review of all deaths, cardiopulmonary arrests in the ED, and all dislodged endotracheal tubes. The plan should review

Table 8. — Standards for Emergency Departments Approved for Pediatrics (EDAP)* (continued)

specific monitors related to care of infants, children, and adolescents in the ED

5.2 A log of all pediatric patients seen in the ED or a method of obtaining these data from the general patient log

*Standards for emergency departments approved for pediatrics (EDAPS). In: *Emergency Medical Services for Children: Development and Integration of Pediatric Emergency Care Into EMS System.* Los Angeles, CA: Los Angeles Pediatric Society, 1984.

†Board-prepared is defined as having successfully completed a board-approved emergency medicine or pediatric residency training program.

‡Full-time is defined as a minimum of 90 hours per month.

EMS Division of the County of Los Angeles Department of Health Services. Guidelines and standards must be adapted to local needs, resources, and the standards of practice in particular communities. The EDAP concept developed in Los Angeles has been implemented with modifications in many other areas of California and in other states.

If we are to assure optimum care, it is important that pediatric patients be offered definitive care in a timely manner. A study in the Chicago area demonstrated that there was an increase in morbidity and mortality of 30% for pediatric patients with head trauma who were in community hospitals and then secondarily transported to a pediatric tertiary care unit. The average delay in definitive care for these patients was 4 hours. A federally funded EMS-C project showed that children who were moderately injured or ill had better outcomes than were predicted by certain physiologic parameters if they received their definitive care in a pediatric center with a pediatric intensive care unit. The patient with the Glasgow Coma Score of 9 might benefit from a pediatric intensive unit and thus a timely transport might be facilitated if the community hospital had a transfer agreement with a pediatric tertiary care center or centers.

In some communities, such as in Los Angeles and the rural areas of California, EMS agencies have developed systems of categorization of hospitals. The hospitals in these areas have differing pediatric capabilities. They are defined according to their ability to care for certain types of patients. The nomenclature is adaptable to other communities. A community hospital with an emergency department approved for pediatrics (EDAP) has verified that it has in place a defined set of equipment and supplies as well as a staff trained in cardiopulmonary resuscitation and in the evaluation of pediatric emergencies. In addition, certain protocols are mandated, including child abuse and neglect policies and transfer policies and procedures. If a community ED has a lower level of care, it may be designated as a Stand-By Emergency Department Approved for Pediatrics. Those rural facilities capable of rendering pediatric care for illness and injury are called Rural Emergency Departments Approved for Pediatrics. Any hospital with secondary or tertiary care capabilities might be termed Local Pediatric Centers, or Pediatric Critical Care Centers. Local Pediatric Centers might have a pediatric observation unit and pediatric ward, while a Pediatric Critical Care Center has the complete spectrum of pediatric subspecialty services, including pediatric trauma.

Categorization of hospitals allows for expedient primary or intrafacility transport to a defined level of care. Models for hospital categorization use different processes to define facilities. Some of these models are shown in Table 9. The child with the femur fracture in the scenario most likely could receive care in a community ED or EDAP. If he had two fractures of major long bones, transfer to a Pediatric Critical Care Center or trauma center might be in order. The child who is post-submersion in the swimming pool is at risk for multisystem disease and would be best cared for in a Pediatric

Table 9. — Implementation Models for Standards

Model	Definition
Categorization	Assessment of a facility based on its ability to manage certain categories of patients. Examples include burn centers, trauma centers, poison centers, level III neonatal intensive care, etc.
Designation	The assigning of responsibility for care of certain categories of patients to specific institutions based on compliance with standards as well as on catchment area or other criteria.
Confirmation	An institution agrees to adopt a set of standards as their own standard on a voluntary basis. They confirm that they have met a standard to care for a certain category of patients.

Critical Care Center that has pediatric nursing and medical specialists.

The evaluation of child abuse, and particularly child sexual abuse, requires a multidisciplinary team, including pediatric behavioral specialists. More will be said in Chapter 9 of this special situation. However, if there is a high index of suspicion, the report can be initiated in the community ED. A referral for a more comprehensive evaluation may be necessary.

Conclusion

Emergency care is best delivered in a vertically integrated system with all members of the community having access to a high quality of care through a 911 system and hospital EDs that are staffed and equipped to manage all age groups. The pediatric equipment and supplies should be organized and readily available. The system may include categorization of facilities but should provide a mechanism for rapid transfer to a higher level of care than might be offered in the community setting. This is best accomplished by predetermined transfer agreements between primary, secondary, and tertiary care facilities. Community hospitals should have policies, procedures, and protocols for pediatric patients in the ED and an area of the ED should be specifically designed to care for children.

Action Points

1. In your community hospitals, determine the degree of formal staff training for pediatric emergencies. If insufficient, suggest enrollment in PALS or APLS.
2. Advocate enrollment of community hospital staffs in CME courses concerning pediatric emergencies. Realize it is difficult to maintain critical pediatric skills.
3. Determine the adequacy of the reference resources available in your community hospital EDs. Suggest texts be purchased that bolster the data base of the emergency providers.
4. Assure that community EDs have equipment appropriate for the care of infants, children, and adolescents.
5. Review ED policies, procedures, and protocols for the care of pediatric emergency patients.

AAP Resources

Appendix E: American Medical Association. Commission on Emergency Medical Services. An Excerpt From "Guidelines for the Categorization of Hospital Emergency Capabilities." *Pediatrics*. 1990;85:879-887

Bibliography

Bushore M: Pediatric emergency care: where do we go from here? A pediatrician's view. *Pediatr Emerg Care*. 1986;2: 258-260

Emergency Medical Services Agency, Health Service Agency, County of Santa Cruz. *Emergency Medical Services for Children*. 1988

Henderson DP, ed. *Emergency Medical Services for Children: Development and Integration of Pediatric Emergency Care into EMS Systems.* Torrance, CA: California EMSC Project; 1989

Holmes MJ, Reyes HM: A critical review of urban pediatric trauma. *J Trauma*. 1984;24:253-255

Los Angeles Pediatric Society: *Information Handbook for Emergency Departments Approved for Pediatrics and Pediatric Critical Care Centers*. Los Angeles, CA: LAPS; 1984

Ludwig S, Fleisher G, Henretig F, Ruddy R: Pediatric training in emergency medicine residency programs. *Ann Emerg Med*. 1982; 11:170-173

Mullner R, Goldberg J: The Illinois trauma system: changes in patient survival patterns following vehicular injuries. *JACEP*. 1977;6:393-396

Pediatric Intensive Care Network of Northern and Central California. *Recommendations for a Regional Pediatric Critical Care System*. Santa Cruz, CA: PICU Network of Northern and Central California; 1988

Pollack MM, Alexander SR, Clarke N, et al. Comparison of tertiary and non-tertiary intensive care: a statewide comparison. *Crit Care Med*. 1991;19:150-159

Ramenofsky M, Luterman A, Quindlen E, Riddick L, Curreri PW. Maximum survival in pediatric trauma: the ideal system. *J Trauma*. 1984;24:818-823

San Francisco Emergency Medical Services Agency, Committee on Pediatric Emergency Medicine. *Standards for Emergency Departments Approved for Pediatrics (EDAP)*. San Francisco, CA: San Francisco Emergency Medical Services Agency; 1990

Seidel JS: A needs assessment of advanced life support and emergency medical services in the pediatric patient: state of the art. *Circulation*. 1986;74(suppl IV):129-133

Seidel JS, Henderson DP, Lewis JB: Emergency medical services and the pediatric patient, III: resources of ambulatory care centers. *Pediatrics*. 1991;88:230-235

Simon JE. Current problems in the emergency management of severe pediatric illness. In: Haller JA, ed. *Emergency Medical Services for Children: Report of the 97th Ross Conference on Pediatric Research*. Columbus, OH: Ross Laboratories; 1989:10-17

State of Hawaii Department of Health: Human Interaction Research Institute, eds. *Emergency Medical Services for Children Innovation Bank 1989*. Honolulu, HI

CHAPTER 7

INTERHOSPITAL TRANSPORT

Cases

A 3-year-old patient with asthma has been treated in your emergency department (ED) for 2 hours and, despite maximal therapy, continues to have significant respiratory distress. In your opinion, the patient needs inpatient treatment at a pediatric tertiary care facility that is 50 miles away.

A 2-year-old girl with epiglottitis has been intubated at your hospital and now needs the services of a pediatric intensive care unit (ICU) that is 70 miles away.

A 7-year-old boy fell off a brick wall and sustained a femur fracture that you believe needs the attention of a pediatric orthopedist who is at a children's hospital 2 hours away by ground transportation.

A 2-month-old girl has presented to your ED in cardiopulmonary arrest of an unknown etiology. After a 30-minute aggressive resuscitation, the patient is stabilized and you decide that she needs pediatric intensive care, available 80 miles away.

Questions

1. What resources are available for transporting these patients for definitive care?
2. Can timely transport to an appropriate hospital reduce disability and total health care cost for critically ill and injured children?
3. What should be the training and composition of the transport teams, and what skills should they have?
4. Under what circumstances are air medical services appropriate?

5. What are the responsibilities of referring and receiving institutions and health care professionals for transported patients?

Key Terms

Prehospital Transport: transportation of the patient from the field (for example, home, physician's office) to the hospital.

Interhospital Transport: interfacility or health care professional transportation of a patient from a referring institution to a receiving hospital.

Secondary Transport: synonymous with interhospital transportation.

The practicing primary care provider will have to transfer a patient to a pediatric tertiary care center for further evaluation and treatment. When the transfer is for subspecialty evaluation of a chronic problem and the patient does not require life support, the parents can take the child for a scheduled appointment. However, when the referral is for an acute or life-threatening illness or injury, the primary care provider must make a decision about the safest and most appropriate method of interfacility transport. This decision should be primarily based on the patient's condition, but it will be affected by many other issues, such as availability of transport resources, weather conditions, cost, and legal issues.

The four options for method of transport include:

1. Transfer by private automobile.
2. Use of a local ambulance service, with or without accompanying support personnel (registered nurse, physician, respiratory therapist) from the referring hospital.
3. Use of a critical care transport team, usually in a helicopter and usually trained in the management of trauma victims and adult cardiac patients.

Table 10. — Advance Preparation for Interhospital Transport

List of pediatric tertiary care facilities with phone numbers

List of transport systems with pediatric capabilities

List (or pack) of equipment and supplies that would be added to usual EMS equipment

Personnel training (PALS, etc)

Administrative protocols

4. Use of a specialized pediatric or neonatal transport team. This option is not available in all areas of the country.

These options, along with their relative indications, advantages, and disadvantages will be discussed in detail in this chapter.

Advance Preparation

It is important that all hospitals have a policy and procedures in place for interfacility transport (Table 10). They should include (1) a list of facilities that are equipped to care for critically ill and injured children (telephone numbers of the facilities should be on the list); (2) a list of transport teams that transport pediatric patients (if different from the teams of the receiving hospitals); (3) the nearest alternate hospital (even if in another state), should the nearest facility not be able to accept a transfer.

If local ambulance transport is an option in your area, advanced preparations are needed. Ambulance personnel should have specific training in pediatric resuscitation. The PALS course is an excellent forum for achieving this training. Clinical training for primary care physicians and others providing acute care is also important. This can be accomplished by allowing emergency medical technicians and physicians time to assist in the care of children in your

ED. Ambulance equipment should be evaluated to assure appropriate pediatric equipment and supplies are available. All ambulances transporting critically ill and injured children should have appropriate equipment and supplies. Registered nurses who may accompany the patient during transport should also have training in pediatric resuscitation. In addition, written protocols for management of potential crises during transport, ie, respiratory failure or arrest, seizure activity, cardiac arrest, etc, also may be helpful.

More extensive equipment may be necessary for physician-accompanied transports or when patients are receiving assisted mechanical ventilation and drug infusion.

In some areas of the country, transfer of patients without insurance coverage is a problem, especially if the nearest available pediatric center is across a state line. Advance preparation for transport, therefore, also must address a variety of administrative issues. This ranges from written, prearranged contracts between the referring and receiving hospitals, to written protocols for the referring physician to follow in order to initiate communication between the administrators of the two hospitals involved. The issue of payment for transport may be separate from that of payment for hospitalization; if this is the case, it should be considered in advance.

The last aspect of advance preparation is to develop an understanding of the legal responsibilities of the parties involved in a transfer. There are variances between states on some of the details. At the federal level, Congress passed the Consolidated Budget Reconciliation Act (COBRA) and the Omnibus Budget Reconciliation Act (OBRA).

COBRA/OBRA Legislation

Congress passed COBRA in 1985 (which included patient transfer requirements) to assure safe patient transfers and to discourage patient "dumping" from hospitals to city- and state-run facilities due to a patient's lack of insurance and/or inability to pay. The legislation required that all patients presenting to an ED receive a screening medical examination; for a transfer to take place, the following must be documented: that the patient's condition is stable, that the receiving hospital has been contacted, that the patient understands the nature of the case, and that there is a physician willing to accept care of the patient. The individual physician who "knowingly" transfers a patient for nonmedical reasons was liable to be sued by the patient or the patient's family, along with the referring institution, for up to $25,000 plus attorney's fees, not including the possibility of a civil suit. The physician can be suspended or expelled from the Medicare program for "knowingly and willfully or negligently" violating federal law.

In 1989 Congress signed into law the Omnibus Budget Reconciliation Act, which became effective on June 1, 1990, and included amendments to the original COBRA legislation referring to patient evaluation and transfer. Parts of the new legislation afford the emergency physician added protection, as opposed to the original COBRA, for certain circumstances encountered in the process of transferring patients. The new laws also place new documentation and reporting requirements on the transferring physician. The OBRA '89 legislation modified the original 1985 COBRA as follows: (1) Hospitals are required to provide a list of on-call physicians who will respond to requests from emergency physicians for inpatient care. Should an on-call physician fail or refuse to respond, the emergency physician will not be liable for an otherwise improper transfer if the physician certifies that the benefit of transfer outweighs the risk to the patient. (2) Emergency physicians are required to report violations of OBRA '89 to the local Medicaid office or to the Inspector General in Washington, DC. "Whistle-blower" protection is afforded, preventing retaliation by hospitals against physicians who report illegal transfers. (3) The provision allowing the individual emergency physician to be sued was deleted. (4) Proof must be provided that a physician "knowingly" transferred an ineligible patient in order for that physician to be liable for civil penalties.

In addition, OBRA '89 requires the following new policies: (1) Hospitals are required to assure that examination and stabilization of patients not be delayed due to determination of payment information. (2) Written consent must be obtained from all patients involved in transfer decisions. A patient is to receive written explanation of risks and benefits of transfer, and effort must be made to have the patients sign the explanations. (3) There is no distinction to be made between "active labor" and an "emergency medical condition." (4) Specialized units and hospitals are required to accept appropriate transfers if they have space and facilities, without regard for ability to pay. Other amendments address record-keeping by hospitals and posting of signs. Potential COBRA violations are investigated by Health Care Financing Committee investigators.

There are two choices in pediatric transport for which inappropriate judgment may be made. The first occurs when the patient is deemed "stable" enough for local ambulance transfer and a crisis occurs for which the crew is untrained, inexperienced, or ill-equipped to handle. A second problem occurs when a trained pediatric team is available for a very critically ill patient, and an "adult" trained team is chosen instead because that team will either arrive at or depart from the referring hospital more quickly. In the first case, the patient's condition may simply deteriorate in a way that could not be anticipated. However, all too often the two mistakes are made because of a misperception that "the faster the patient is on the way (or gone from the ED) the better." There is no evidence that the speed of transfer, regardless of level of care en route, is beneficial to the pediatric patient. Intuitively, this may be the case for a small percentage of patients such as those with immediate surgical emergencies (ie, those who need the physical facilities of the receiving hospital). For the vast majority of pediatric patients, level of care during transfer will be more important. Again, the referring hospital is legally responsible for assuring that the level of care is appropriate.

Communication With the Receiving Hospital

The initial call to transfer a patient should be from physician to physician. The referring physician should have the patient's chart available at the time of the call in order to be able to provide specific details about vital signs, fluids administered, timing of events, etc. In a crisis situation, a brief history of the illness/injury, interventions performed, and current clinical status will be sufficient information to allow for treatment recommendations and a decision about method of transport. Document the name of the accepting physician, the accepting hospital, and any advice received. If a transport team from the receiving hospital is to be used, the accepting physician will activate the system and call back later if further information is needed or there are any other interventions to recommend.

The referring physician can call the receiving hospital at any time during the transfer process if the patient's condition changes or any further suggestions for patient management are needed. Nurse-to-nurse communication from the referring to the referral hospital also should be encouraged. Nursing personnel from either hospital should feel free to request or provide updates on the patient's status. If a method of transport is chosen that does not involve the receiving hospital's transport team, a report should be called to that hospital immediately prior to the patient's departure. This report includes the patient's most recent vital signs, current clinical status, and estimated time of arrival at the receiving hospital. The tertiary care center that accepts the patient has a responsibility to provide accessible telephone advice, and the transferring hospital has a responsibility to try to provide reasonable information needed to offer such advice. The referring physician has the greatest legal responsibility for the choice of transport mode, but the decision should be a joint one between the referring and receiving physicians. If both parties agree on a method of transport, they will share some level of legal responsibility for adverse events during transfer. The receiving physician has to make a determination without the advantage of examining the patient, and the referring physician often has to make a decision without the benefit of having experience with large numbers of critically ill children. This can be an uncomfortable situation from both sides, and it is important to remember that the goal is to work together in the best interest of the child.

Another part of the communication process is the transfer of copies of all records, laboratory results, and x-rays with the patient. Pending results at the time of departure should be noted, along with a telephone number to call for results.

Options for Interhospital Transport

Three types of medically equipped vehicles are used for interfacility patient transport. Ground ambulance transport is by far the most common. For critically ill patients or those who must be transferred long distances, helicopters and fixed-wing aircraft are also used. Ideally, a region will be served by teams with access to all three types of vehicles. In practice, however, access is often limited to one or two types of vehicles, especially for dedicated pediatric and neonatal teams.

Ground ambulances are relatively inexpensive and safe. They can easily be stopped, if necessary, for clinical assessment or intervention (ie, to replace an IV, decide if an endotracheal tube is dislodged, or to place a chest tube). This form of transport can be slow, especially in major cities with dense traffic. Helicopters are fast and do not encounter traffic problems. However, they are expensive and it is difficult to monitor patients or to perform procedures in transit. Safety concerns for crew and patient are legitimate concerns that have recently received a great deal of attention. Fixed-wing aircraft are only an option for long-distance transport. Their cost is comparable to that of helicopter transport. Monitoring and interventions are easier than in a helicopter but more difficult than in a ground ambulance. Safety is less of a concern than for helicopters, largely because of sophisticated instruments and the controlled environment of airports.

Private Automobile

The indications for interfacility transport of a sick child via the parent's car are limited to those patients with very chronic, mild, or stable illnesses who have virtually no chance of their conditions deteriorating during the transfer time. The main advantage of this form of transport is the lowered cost. In addition, availability of transport resources is maintained (ie, if you are not using the transport system, it remains available for another patient).

The disadvantage of transport by private car is total loss of control of the patient, and medical intervention is impossible. Additionally, the referring physician may assume the family is going directly to the other hospital, when in fact they may first go home or elsewhere, or even decide that the child looks better and does not need to go at all. In cases in which the physician strongly believes that the patient needs tertiary evaluation and care but is unsure of the family's commitment to seek that care, local ambulance transport may be more appropriate. In none of the four case scenarios would transportation by the family be a tenable option.

Local Ambulance

There are two situations in which it is appropriate to use a local ambulance. The first is for the patient who is very stable, preferably not traveling a long distance, but who needs a minor level of medical care (ie, maintenance of an IV, low level oxygen therapy); assurance of rapid, direct transport to the receiving hospital; or the benefit of a stretcher (ie, isolated femur fracture). Availability of the appropriate-sized resuscitation equipment for the patient's age should be verified prior to transport. Remember to make sure that the ambulance has equipment, supplies, and travel personnel appropriate for the level of care required by the patient. Studies have shown that EMT training in pediatric emergency care often is limited and that sophisticated advanced life support interventions may not always be possible using standard EMT-attended ambulance transport. The 7-year-old child in our scenario with an isolated femur fracture, if appropriately evaluated and stabilized at the hospital, could be transported by a local ambulance. The child's fracture can be appropriately immobilized and the patient can be comfortable during a ride in the ambulance. He should not be given pain control medication, which could cause respiratory depression during transport.

An added level of care can be provided by sending a skilled nurse from the referring hospital in the ambulance with the patient. Vital signs can be monitored and interpreted more frequently. However, careful consideration must be given to the situation and to the pediatric skills of the individual nurse. Nurses in many hospitals that refer pediatric patients have little experience themselves in pediatric crises. Expectations for care needed during transfer should not exceed the skills that would normally be provided by that nurse, unsupervised, in the referring hospital. "It's OK, I'm sending a nurse along" won't cover the level of care needed for a critically ill child.

The second situation in which use of a local ambulance is indicated is for the patient who needs the immediate physical facilities of the receiving hospital, and no faster way of arriving there is available. Examples of this scenario include cases of patients with an immediate need for surgical intervention (ie, epidural hematoma, certain forms of major trauma) for whom air transport is not available (due to lack of resources or to weather). Critically ill or injured persons who require ground transport by a local ambulance should always be accompanied by a physician. This is the situation in which preplanned equipment lists and/or packs will reduce the stress of getting ready to leave and will prevent forgetting a crucial medication or instrument.

The greatest advantage of local ambulance transport is lowered cost as compared with other means of transportation. Other advantages include assurance of timely transfer and maintenance of some level of control over care (depending on accompanying personnel and protocols).

One disadvantage in using ambulance transport involves loss of local resources. A rural region may have a large geographic area covered by a single ambulance service. Loss of that resource for several hours to care for a single patient may be unacceptable if it leaves a particular region without an ambulance. Similarly, a community hospital may have a single physician on duty in the ED. It is not likely that person can leave the area for a prolonged period of time.

For a critically ill child, with a high potential to have their condition deteriorate during transfer, the disadvantages of a local ambulance transport far outweigh the advantages. Thus the children in the scenarios with status asthmaticus, epiglottitis, and cardiopulmonary arrest are not candidates for such transportation. As previously discussed, the usual ambulance personnel are neither trained nor equipped to manage these children who are being transferred because of need for an ICU environment.

This is especially true if that transfer is over a long distance. The addition of a nurse to the ambulance crew also may not raise the level of care to the necessary point and a physician may be required to accompany the patient. Addition of the referring physician to a local ambulance to care for the patient en route also does not assure optimum care if the physician is uncomfortable with management of the child's problem, the equipment being used, or therapy initiated. If the transfer is partly requested because the physician has not cared for a patient with the particular illness for a long time and believes the patient's interests will be better served by someone with more frequent experience, another means of transportation such as a transportation team should be used.

Transport Teams

Transport teams may serve a particular region. They may be capable of ground as well as air transportation. They are typically trained and experienced in the care of trauma and adult cardiac patients. Transport team members are usually trained or based in the ED (or sometimes the ICU) of the hospital that runs the service. A primary care provider seeking transportation of a critical pediatric patient needs to know the following: does the base hospital treat critically ill children, thus giving team members ongoing pediatric experience? Or do they refer their sickest children to the tertiary care center your patient is going to? What specific pediatric training and experience are required of team members? Some systems have extensive programs designed to orient the team to pediatric care, while others offer little more than the option to take the PALS course. What percentage of transports are for children? If the answer is less than 10% to 20% and the hospital refers critically ill children, it is unlikely that the team will be comfortable or experienced in pediatric care. Is a physician part of the flight team? Many broad-based systems use a nurse-nurse or nurse-paramedic team.

Currently that system seems to work well for most adult patients. At this time, scientific data are inconclusive as to whether a physician is beneficial. More than 90% of pediatric transport teams, other than neonatal, include a physician. If there is no physician on the team and the team does not have much pediatric experience, one should seriously consider whether that team will be able to manage the patient optimally in transit.

If a region is served by a pediatric or neonatal transport system that has access to ground and air transportation, utilization of their services may be preferable to an adult-oriented transport team. The only exception is when the pediatric team is not available.

Helicopter transfers may be preferred over a pediatric ground transport system when there is a life-threatening condition such as multiple trauma, and rapid transport for definitive care is vital. Some pediatric teams are staffed by pediatric residents who may not have extensive experience with trauma patients. While the adult-trained team may be inexperienced with children, they will have a great deal of experience with victims of multiple trauma.

The advantage of the broad-based team lies entirely in the speed of arrival at the receiving hospital. This is not to be confused with speed of delivery of sophisticated pediatric care to the patient. A pediatric team using ground transportation can often arrive to begin pediatric intensive care within the same time frame of a round-trip helicopter ride. However, the patient will be maintained in a stable environment with all of the resources of the referring hospital instead of in a moving vehicle in the air. Patient monitoring is difficult in a helicopter because of noise and vibrations. The effect is enhanced for small patients (ie, if it is difficult to hear an adult's breath sounds in a helicopter, it is impossible to hear an infant's). For this reason, some pediatric transport systems with access to a helicopter choose often to travel by ground anyway.

Total reliance on helicopter transport for all critical patients will have the added disadvantage of inability to transport during the 10% to 20% of the time that helicopters are unable to fly due to adverse weather conditions.

Dedicated Pediatric or Neonatal Transport Team

When available in a given region, a pediatric team should be used for the transfer of a child who is too unstable or potentially unstable for transfer via local ambulance. There are currently no scoring systems or specific criteria that have been proven to predict need for a transport team. Broad recommendations for use of a pediatric transport team include the following transfer situations:

1. Any patient for whom ICU admission is anticipated at the receiving hospital.

2. Patients with respiratory distress that may progress during the time of transfer, ie, a patient with asthma or croup who may not need ICU admission but whose condition may worsen enough to need intervention during an hour-long ride.

3. Patients with a recent life-threatening event, although they are stable at the time of transfer. This would include neonates with a history of significant apnea and any patient who has required aggressive resuscitation (ie, seizure with apnea, shock), because whatever happened before could happen again.

The advantages of a pediatric team include the high level of training and experience in pediatric critical care, use of portable monitors designed for small patients, availability of equipment and medications for a wide range of ages, and continuity of care when the receiving hospital reaches out to assume and maintain care of the patient during transfer.

The disadvantages of pediatric teams are their possible lack of access to all three types of transport vehicles, possible lack of experience with multiple trauma, and lack of availability of these teams in certain regions. Turning to our illustrative cases, the 3-year-old boy with asthma has been treated in an ED that is 1 hour's drive from the tertiary care center. He has required multiple aerosolized bronchodilators, an aminophylline infusion, and a steroid bolus. He is awake and alert. Arterial blood gas determination after therapy shows the following values: pH, 7.35; pCO_2, 40 mm Hg; and pO_2, 150 mm Hg while receiving 4 L/minute of oxygen via face mask. He is to be transferred because the referring hospital cannot manage a pediatric inpatient with significant respiratory distress. For the transportation the physician must choose between a local ambulance and a critical care transport team. In this case, an ambulance alone or with a nurse would not be appropriate because the patient has the possibility of respiratory failure. If a physician is available to go and has the necessary equipment and skills for intubation of a 3-year-old, that method of transport would be fine. If not, and a pediatric team is available, that would be the best choice (whether they travel by ground or by air).

The 2-year-old girl with epiglottitis has already been intubated and is in an ED 1 hour away from the receiving hospital. She was in significant distress on presentation, but she is now breathing easily with her endotracheal tube in place. She is sedated to prevent agitation. Her physician wishes to transfer her. The choice of transportation is an adult-trained transport team by helicopter or a pediatric transport team by ground. The pediatric team would be the most appropriate for patient management, but there is concern about transport time. If a helicopter is available, it takes 10 minutes to lift off, 20 minutes of flight time, 15 minutes in the referring hospital, and 20 minutes of flight time back. The patient will receive pediatric intensive care after 1 hour and 5 minutes. If the pediatric team is able to depart from their hospital within 15 to 30 minutes, the patient will receive pediatric intensive care within 1 hour and 30 minutes.

With the second choice, the patient is in the best environment with the best team to perform reintubation should it become necessary during transport. Despite the fact that the referring hospital would have to maintain the patient for an hour and a half as opposed to 30 minutes, the patient's interest may best be served by use of the pediatric team by ground.

The 2-month-old girl who presented in cardiopulmonary arrest to an adult ED 1½ hours from a tertiary care center has been resuscitated. At the time of the call for transfer, she is receiving a dopamine infusion. She is intubated and ventilated. She has received antibiotics and she is receiving a continuous infusion of sodium bicarbonate. Her blood pressure is normal for patients her age receiving dopamine.

A broad-based helicopter team is available, as well as a pediatric transport team that would travel by ground. The helicopter team does not routinely care for children, especially infants of this age. Again, although the helicopter can probably arrive in about 45 minutes, the pediatric team is more appropriate. This patient has a good chance for further cardiovascular instability and will need to remain in a stable environment until a team highly experienced and skilled in pediatric intensive care can take over patient management.

Preparing for Arrival of a Transport Team

When a transport team from another hospital is used, the referring hospital can do a great deal to assist in the efficient, timely transfer of the patient. Ask what form of consent to transport is required by the team. Some teams operate with an understanding of implied consent and some transport as a life-threatening emergency without

Table 11. — Preparing for the Transport Team

Copy all records and radiographs
Obtain transport consent
Secure all lines and tubes
Stabilize C-spine and fractures, if appropriate
Prepare blood products, if appropriate
Remain at bedside and/or be available for consultation

formal consent. If at all possible, written consent to transport should be obtained from the patient's legal guardian. Some transport teams will request that the parents remain present at the hospital to give consent directly to the team. This is often because the team needs access to the parents for details of the patient's past medical history and current condition. Too frequently the parents leave the referring hospital prior to arrival of the team but do not arrive at the receiving hospital until several hours after the patient, causing a significant void in the information needed to care for the child.

In-hospital turnaround time for the transport team can be significantly reduced by advance preparation for transport by the referring hospital (Table 11). Lines and tubes will often need additional stabilization prior to patient transfer. A frequent adverse event during transport is loss of a line or tube because it was not secured adequately for a moving, vibrating environment. The referring hospital can secure all tubes and lines prior to the arrival of the transport team and decrease the time the team spends before departure. In addition, the cervical spine and any fractured bones may need to be stabilized in a secure fashion. Copies of the patient's chart and x-rays should be made prior to arrival of the team. If the patient might need blood products during transport, arrange in advance to obtain a supply to send with the team. In general, transfer will be more efficient if the referring hospital anticipates what the team will need and takes care of some of the details in advance.

Follow-up After Transportation

Many transport teams will either provide an evaluation form for the referring hospital or will contact the referring physician after the transport is completed to learn if there were any problems. If this is not done, the referring physician can contact the medical director of the transport system for information or discussion of the transport of a particular patient.

If the transport team comes from the receiving hospital, team members can tell the referring physician who the attending physician will be at the tertiary care center. In many cases, the transport team is independent of the receiving hospital. Therefore, the transport team members, or even the transport medical director, may not know details about the patient's progress, condition, or prognosis if called the next day.

The attending physician at the tertiary care center is responsible for providing follow-up on the ongoing condition of the patient and the ultimate outcome of the patient's hospitalization. This information may be communicated to the patient's primary care physician or other referring health care provider such as the emergency medicine physician.

Action Items

1. Prepare and post in your office a list of facilities that care for critically ill and injured children. Include their telephone numbers.
2. Suggest adequate training for local ambulance personnel who transport critically ill or injured children.
3. Assure that pediatric equipment and supplies are available by your local ambulance service.

4. Physicians should know how the COBRA and OBRA legislations relate to patient transfer.
5. Know the pediatric capabilities of your region's broad-based dedicated transport team.
6. Learn how to prepare a critical pediatric patient while awaiting transport to another hospital facility.

AAP Resources

American Academy of Pediatrics, Task Force on Interhospital Transport. Guidelines for air and ground transport of pediatric patients (revision of 1986 Policy Statement under development).

Bibliography

American Academy of Pediatrics, Committee on Hospital Care. Guidelines for air and ground transportation of pediatric patients. *Pediatrics*. 1986;78:943-950

Baker MD, Ludwig S. Pediatric emergency transport and the private practitioner. *Pediatrics*. 1991;88:691-695

Barkin RM, ed. Pediatrics in the emergency medical services system. *Pediatr Emerg Care*. 1990:6:72-77

Day S, McCloskey K, Orr R, Bolte R, Notterman D, Hackel A. Pediatric interhospital critical care transport: consensus of a national leadership conference. *Pediatrics*. 1991;88:696-704

Hunt RC, Bryan DM, Brinkley VS, Whitley TW, Benson NH. Inability to assess breath sounds during air medical transport by helicopter. *JAMA*. 1991;265:1982-1984

McCloskey KA, Orr RA. Pediatric transport issues in emergency medicine. *Emerg Med Clin North Am*. 1991;9:475-489

Macnab AJ. Optimal escort for interhospital transport of pediatric emergencies. *J Trauma*. 1991;31:205-209

Seidel JS. Emergency medical services and the pediatric patient: are the needs being met? II: training and equipping emergency medical services providers for pediatric emergencies. *Pediatrics*. 1986;78:808-812

Seidel JS, Hornbein M, Yoshiyama K, Kuznets D, Finklestein JZ, St Geme JW, Jr. Emergency medical services and the pediatric patient: are the needs being met? *Pediatrics*. 1984;73:769-772

Yamamoto LG, Wiebe RA, Maiava DM, Merry CJ. A one-year series of pediatric prehospital care. I: ambulance runs. II: prehospital communication. III: interhospital transport services. *Pediatr Emerg Care*. 1991;7:206-214

CHAPTER 8

THE REFERRAL HOSPITAL

Case

You are requested to consult on a 3-year-old patient who has presented to a rural hospital. The child has experienced polydipsia, polyuria, and weight loss for 1 week. The treating physician has established a diagnosis of diabetes mellitus. The child is alert, verbal, and is mildly ketonemic. The parents are uninsured and have limited access to transportation.

Questions

1. How can the pediatrician establish a link with a facility to move an ill or injured child safely to a secondary or tertiary care center?
2. How can a pediatrician match the high-risk and critical patient's needs with proper facilities providing specialized care?
3. What are the potential advantages of transportation agreements?

Key Terms

Transfer Agreement: An agreement that delineates the responsibilities of both the referring and referral hospitals.

The referral hospital is a vital component of an Emergency Medical Services System for Children. Choice of referral hospital must be well defined. Access to that hospital must be prompt. Communications with that referral hospital should be smooth and ongoing rather than limited to those times surrounding an imminent transfer.

Choice of Referral Hospital

The availability of appropriate medical resources for the child in need of transfer should be the primary guide to the choice of referral hospital. The AMA has published "Guidelines for the Categorization of Hospital Emergency Capabilities." The Academy has endorsed the section in these "Guidelines" that addresses pediatric emergency capabilities (Appendix E). These guidelines may be used by regional and state organizations to define the capabilities of referral hospitals.

Other factors that need to be considered in the choice of a referral hospital include current utilization of a hospital's resources, distance and transport time, mode of transport, and last, but by no means least, a practitioner's firsthand knowledge of the actual resources of a given referral hospital.

Two additional factors, politics and economics, should have no role in the choice of referral hospital. Local politics, that is the desire to support one hospital versus another or one receiving physician versus another, should not be played out at the expense of appropriate care for the individual patient. Similarly, it is the position of the Academy that all children have the right to be referred to the level of care commensurate with their medical problems regardless of their third-party payor status. This position has been expanded in the statement of the Academy entitled "Access to Emergency Medical Care" (see Appendix J).

Transfer Agreements

The recommended mechanism for guaranteeing prompt access to a referral hospital appropriate for a given patient is a transfer agreement. This agreement delineates the responsibilities of the referring and referral hospital and their respective medical staffs. It clarifies issues of access, communication, liability, and timing. It may be invoked to speed a particular transfer as well as to review the management of a series of transfers. Above all, it is an agreement developed in the "light of day" rather than in the middle of a battle to save a child's life. A transfer agreement prototype is illustrated in Appendix K. Its individual components will be briefly discussed.

Transfer Decision. In the transfer agreement prototype in Appendix K, item 1 establishes that the decision to transfer to the referral hospital is a shared decision. Only the referring hospital can determine if the patient's needs exceed its resources. Only the receiving hospital can determine if current utilization of its resources is at a level that will accommodate the patient to be transferred. Item 3 of the transfer document also enables the referral hospital to prevent referrals of patients for which it lacks appropriate specialty resources.

Referring Hospital Responsibilities

In the transfer agreement (prototype in Appendix K), item 2 delineates the responsibilities of the referring hospital, including obtaining informed consent, providing appropriate medical documentation, and consulting regarding mode of transport. Most importantly, items 4 and 6 clearly seek to place liability for the patient's care on the referring hospital's shoulders until a physician from the referral hospital is able to assume bedside care. Despite this provision, however, the referral hospital, by virtue of the telephone advice it provides, should still regard itself as "at risk" from the moment of contact with the referring hospital. Careful documentation and conservative advice that consistently acknowledge the limits of medical advice without the benefit of bedside examination are the referral hospital's best protection.

Transport Costs

Transport costs may be handled in many ways. The provision in this sample agreement has the disadvantage that transport services may reject the transport for fear of lack of remuneration. Another option is to place the fiscal responsibility on the referring hospital. If the referring hospital would accept this provision, it might both speed the transport and guarantee a higher level of transport sophistication.

Communication

Item 9 in the prototype agreement stipulates that communication will be physician to physician and nurse to nurse. Also, by providing a single mechanism for referral, better record-keeping regarding referrals is guaranteed. Item 10 makes it clear that the referral hospital has a responsibility to provide ongoing communication back to the referring hospital.

Criteria for Referral/Acceptance

Unfortunately, a patient's third-party funding does play a role in hospitals' decisions to transfer and to accept transferred patients. Financial matters may be raised as in the above scenario for the uninsured patient. One of the prime advantages of a transfer agreement is that it allows hospitals to discuss this issue openly across a conference table rather than serendipitously as part of a medical communication regarding the care and transfer of a sick child. Though seemingly difficult to enforce, these provisions place each hospital on notice that its behavior vis-à-vis this issue is subject to monitoring and review. This provision also gives each hospital the authority to demand that its own medical staff deals with the other hospital and its medical staff in a uniform and predictable fashion.

Issues Concerning Communications

Issues concerning communications beyond those discussed in the sample transfer agreement warrant some discussion. Specifically, communications between the referring and referral hospital should not be limited to communications surrounding an individual patient transfer. The continuing medical education programs, protected quality assurance communications, and ongoing review of the transfer agreement and compliance with that agreement should be formalized. Traditionally, the first item, CME programs, has been addressed with a "come to the Mecca" approach. The other items generally do not occur or do so only around a crisis. A portion of the referral hospital's CME program should be shared with the referring hospital where broader participation may be achieved and care recommendations can be made in the context of a referring hospital's actual resources. Quality assurance communications should occur *regularly* rather than simply as a reaction to a difficult case. This allows for positive as well as critical feedback. When critical feedback is necessary (in either direction), the lines of communication will be open and, hopefully, receptive.

Finally, the transfer agreement should be reviewed periodically in the light of accumulated data rather than simply in reaction to a specific transfer. Among other considerations, this alerts both institutions that the transfer agreement exists and compliance with its provisions is being monitored. It also allows for the prompt recognition of the need to change selected provisions of the agreement in response to changing resources or other factors.

Reverse Referral

The referral hospital has the right to expect that the referring hospital will accept a patient back to its facility when that patient's care needs can be met by the resources of that hospital. A provision addressing this issue may be incorporated into the original transfer agreement.

Summary

The referral hospital is both a valuable and vulnerable resource. Because minutes are crucial in the fight to care for a desperately ill child, access to the referral hospital's valuable resources must be prompt. Offering such access, however, renders the referral hospital vulnerable to "economic transfers." The solution to this dilemma is a well-conceived transfer agreement developed in the board room rather than negotiated between emergency departments, monitored closely, and enriched by ongoing dialogue between the referring and referral hospitals.

Action Points

1. Within a geographic locale, refer patients to an appropriate facility that matches the needs of the patient based on your knowledge of the capabilities of equally equipped facilities.

2. Establish a pattern of referral such that persons who have previously undergone specialized treatment can receive continuity of care.

3. Establish and update referral agreements between hospital facilities and your community.

Bibliography

Sacchetti A, Carraccio C, Warden T, Gazak S. Community hospital management of pediatric emergencies: implications for pediatric emergency medical services. *Am J Emerg Med.* 1986;4:10-13

Simon J. Optimizing pediatric emergency care with suboptimal resources. In: Harwood-Nuss A, Luten R, eds. *Problems in Pediatric Emergency Medicine.* New York, NY: Churchill Livingstone Inc; 1988:29-44

Simon JE, Smookler S, Guy B. A regionalized approach to pediatric emergency care. *Pediatr Clin North Am.* 1981;28: 677-687

CHAPTER 9

PLANNING FOR SPECIAL SITUATIONS

Cases

A local school bus is involved in a crash at a train crossing.

A 14-year-old boy presents to your office unaccompanied by a parent with complaints of a penile discharge.

You are consulted by the local emergency department (ED) concerning an 18-month-old child who is brought in by the babysitter. Concerns are expressed due to the child's multiple bruises.

A mother calls the office saying her 16-year-old daughter has locked herself in the bathroom and taken a number of pills.

A local ED calls and says one of your 7-month-old patients had a cardiac arrest at home and could not be revived.

These are but a few examples of situations in emergency medical services that require special planning.

Questions

1. What advance preparations are necessary on the part of the primary care provider to care for special pediatric situations successfully?

2. What roles must the primary care provider assume at times of family crisis, including such events as abuse, neglect, intoxication, suicidal behavior, and unexpected pediatric death?

Key Terms

Emergency: Any condition that requires immediate medical attention in the opinion of the patient, family, or whoever assumes the responsibility of bringing the patient to the attention of the physician.

True Emergency: Any condition clinically determined to require immediate medical care. Conditions that are a threat to the patient's health are sufficient to be considered true emergency; life and limb need not be threatened.

Emergent: A medical condition that requires immediate medical attention; delay may be harmful to the patient and the disorder is acute and potentially threatens life or function.

Urgent: A medical condition that requires attention within a few hours and will be of danger if not attended to within that time frame; disorder is acute but not necessarily severe.

In these situations the goals for preparedness are (1) the establishment of written policies and procedures that cover these events and (2) compliance with the Joint Commission for the Accreditation of Healthcare Organizations (JCAHO) standards for emergency services. Planning for these special situations also affects system design. For example, in each ED, an area to be used as a parent's room or quiet room where the family may wait in privacy or consult with the physician should be designated. In this chapter examples of these special situations will be listed, emphasizing guidelines useful for the physician who is responsible for the establishment of policy.

Mass Casualty/Disaster Plan

A mass casualty/disaster plan should be designed to manage the consequences of natural disasters or other emergencies in which multiple casualties threaten to disrupt the hospitals' ability to provide care and treatment. The JCAHO *Accreditation Manual for Hospitals* outlines specific standards for emergency preparedness and serves as a valuable resource for planning. Model systems have been proposed by organizations such as the American College of Surgeons Committee on Trauma and the American College of Emergency Physicians.

The first step in mass casualty/disaster planning is to contact your local or state Department of Health or American Academy of Pediatrics Chapter and find out if there is a state, regional, or local plan in effect. It is important that the hospital's plan be written as a part of a coordinated community-wide effort. Physicians with an interest in child health should play a particular role in the review of community and hospital plans to ascertain pediatric components that address the special needs of children. The statewide or community plan should contain provisions for scene triage that recognize and utilize pediatric resources such as EDs, burn units, trauma centers, and intensive care units. The hospital plan should contain pediatric components for notification of parents, possible transfer to other special resource facilities, and procedures for discharge. Other components of the plan should include the following.

1. Specific guidelines for activation of the plan. This should include information about who will have the authority to activate the plan, under what circumstances they should be instructed to activate, and how the hospital will implement the plan. Implementation of the plan should include specific procedures for notification of additional or key personnel, establishment of command post, and a system for patient identification and record-keeping. Phone lists are frequently used as a method for contacting key personnel. If this system is used, the lists must be updated on at least a yearly basis. A workable plan for patient identification and record-keeping is essential. One method is to start with a triage log that assigns a number along with a folder containing identically numbered wristbands, requisitions, a triage tag, and other medical records to the patient on arrival. The triage tag is used to track the patient's movement through the hospital system, while the medical record folder stays with the patient throughout his or her hospital stay.

2. Provisions must be made for the effective use of space, the procurement of additional supplies, the establishment of efficient communication between heavily used areas of the hospital, and increased security.

3. Provisions must be made for the management of staff, including distribution and assignment of responsibilities and functions.

4. Provisions must be made for the management of patients, including triage, scheduling of services, control of patient information, notification of parents, admission, transfer, and discharge. Pediatric disasters will require greater manpower needs and space for extended family members.

5. Provisions must be made for the management of deceased patients.

6. The staff must be trained to understand the overall plan and the function of their roles during emergencies.

7. The plan and personnel should be tested through semiannual implementations, either in response to an actual mass casualty or as part of a planned drill, which will include a written evaluation of the performance of the emergency department.

It is appropriate for primary care providers to know both their community's response and their individual responsibilities for children involved in a mass casualty such as the bus/train collision depicted in the case scenario.

Unaccompanied Minor Requiring Care

Standards of the JCAHO require that EDs have written policies and procedures for the provision of care to unaccompanied minors. Unfortunately, surveys have noted as many as 14% of EDs reporting no written policy in effect. Physicians should not only check local EDs to make sure

Table 12. — Examples of Emancipated Minor*

Married (past or present)

High school graduate

Pregnant (past or present)

Self-supporting

Serving in armed forces

Living independently

Runaways

Abandoned minors

*Adapted from Selbst SM. Treating minors without their parents. *Pediatr Emerg Care.* 1985; 1:168-173, with permission.

a written policy is in effect but prepare written guidelines for their offices. The first step in preparing a policy is to ascertain the provisions of your state's law with regard to the mature minor doctrine and/or the definition of an emancipated minor. Most states recognize an emancipated minor as one who can seek and receive medical attention without parental consent (Appendix L). State and local medical societies are usually very helpful in the process of obtaining copies of the law. Most states have laws that permit treatment of minors either as an emancipated minor or in selected cases without parental consent. Usually the definition of an emancipated minor includes those who have been married or pregnant, graduated from high school, or are otherwise independent of parental care or control (Table 12). Examples of selected instances in which it is possible for a minor to provide consent on her or his own would include the treatment of venereal disease, pregnancy, or for alcohol or substance abuse (Table 13). The mature minor doctrine currently in effect in 22 states gives adolescents more than 14 or 15 years old the right to consent to all needed medical care. If the minor understands the nature and risks of the proposed treatment, then he or she may consent to care. The age and maturity

Table 13. — Examples of Medical Conditions Not Requiring Parental Consent*

Any medical emergency
Venereal disease
Pregnancy
Contraceptive services
Drug or alcohol abuse services
Abortion

*From Selbst SM. Treating minors without their parents. *Pediatr Emerg Care.* 1985;1:168-173, with permission.

of the adolescent, nature of the illness, and risks of therapy should be considered when making the decision to treat before obtaining parental consent. When possible, the mature minor should be asked to sign a consent form for needed emergency procedures in the absence of a parent, as would be done for an adult.

Treatment without parental consent in all states is generally permissible in an emergency situation. The definition of an emergency varies depending on the jurisdiction and, again, your local laws should be ascertained. In most instances an emergency can be defined as any condition that is a threat to the health of the child and requires prompt treatment. It is not limited to life- or limb-threatening illness. Although it is important to be familiar with the law, these statutes are frequently ambiguous and, therefore, subject to a great deal of interpretation. This should prompt the physician to clearly document in the medical record all attempts to contact the parent for consent when decisions are made for immediate treatment. In cases in which invasive procedures are required, it is helpful to document a second opinion agreeing with the necessity of the procedure.

In the absence of an emergency, a careful evaluation of the patient's condition is still warranted. *Although the unauthorized treatment of a patient legally constitutes battery, failure to evaluate and treat probably carries greater risk for negligence.* In the situation described above of a minor who is brought for care by someone other than the parent or guardian, similar principles apply. The caretaker may be considered to be acting in loco parentis. The physician should be careful to evaluate and act in the best interest of the child while documenting on the medical record special concerns or circumstances. The response is especially critical if a child accompanied by someone other than the parent or legal guardian is brought to see a physician for evaluation of suspected abuse or neglect.

Child Abuse and Sexual Assault

Child abuse may be subdivided into four categories to include (1) physical abuse, (2) sexual abuse, (3) emotional abuse, and (4) neglect. Established protocols and procedures for the office and ED direct the physician in the evaluation and management of these cases. Although community resources differ considerably, many metropolitan areas have special programs or facilities that can assist the physician in the development of protocols. Optimal evaluation and management are best performed in a regional center, capable of providing comprehensive services in a nonthreatening environment. Referral to the ED should be reserved for cases of acute injury. A list of Child Abuse and Sexual Assault Centers compiled by the Section on Child Abuse and Neglect of the Academy is provided in Appendix M. The goals of the protocol should be: (1) Alert ED or office personnel to the presenting signs and symptoms of child abuse (Table 14). (2) Aid the physician in obtaining pertinent information from the history and physical examination. (3) Set criteria for obtaining and the proper handling and transport of forensic specimens, laboratory tests, radiologic studies, and photographs (Table 15). (4) Provide that the medical record carefully

Table 14. — Indicators of Abuse*

Historical Indicators of Abuse

 Is the history one of inflicted injury?

 Is there an absence of history, a "magical" injury?

 Could the injury have been avoided by better care and supervision?

 Are there inconsistencies or changes in the history?

 Is there a history of repeated injury or hospitalizations?

 Was there a delay in seeking medical care?

 Does the history overestimate or underestimate the injury?

 Is there a past medical history of prematurity, failure to thrive, failure to receive adequate medical care such as immunization?

Physical Indicators of Abuse

 Does injury match the history of injury?

 Are there pathognomonic injuries such as looped wire marks, cigarette burns, etc?

 Are there multiple injuries?

 Are the injuries at various stages of healing?

 Are there different injury forms, for example, burns and fractures?

 Is there evidence of overall poor care?

 Has poisoning been documented in a young child?

 Is there evidence of failure to thrive without a history of symptoms or physical findings?

 Are there any visual or unexplained physical findings?

*From Ludwig S. Child abuse. In: Fleisher GR, Ludwig S, eds. *Textbook of Pediatric Emergency Medicine.* 2nd ed. Baltimore, MD: Williams & Wilkins Co; 1988: chap 81, with permission.

documents the history, physical examination, evaluation, and the treatment given. (5) Provide for the prompt reporting of the incident to the proper authorities. (6) Provide for immediate and follow-up consultation and counseling with special resource personnel such as social service or child psychiatry. A copy of the state Child Abuse Law should be included with the written policy. Separate protocols should be developed for physical abuse and sexual abuse. In both instances it is helpful to include standard line drawings of the body and genitalia to aid in the

Table 15. — Laboratory and Radiographic Indicators of Abuse*

Studies	Indication
Hematologic	
Prothrombin time	Bleeding disorders
Partial thromboplastin time	Bleeding disorders
Platelet count	Bleeding disorders
Complete blood count including red blood cell indices	Blood loss, nutritional anemia
Biochemical	
Blood urea nitrogen	Dehydration
Creatine phosphokinase	Muscle injury
Amylase	Abdominal trauma
Electrolytes, osmolality: Calcium, phosphorous/ alkaline phosphatase	Dehydration, water intoxication, bone disease
Toxicology screen	Poisoning
Urine	
Specific gravity	Dehydration
Blood	Renal or genital trauma
Ferric chloride	Poisoning
Radiographic	
Skeletal survey for trauma	Periosteal elevation
Bone scan	Subperiosteal hemorrhage
	Metaphyseal chip fractures
	Epiphyseal separation
	Spiral fractures in nonambulatory patients
	Fractures in various stages of healing
	Rib fractures
	Unusual fractures
Upper gastrointestinal series	Duodenal hematoma
Computerized tomography scan	Head trauma, shaking injury

*From Ludwig S. Child abuse. In: Fleisher GR, Ludwig S, eds. *Textbook of Pediatric Emergency Medicine.* 2nd ed. Baltimore, MD: Williams & Wilkins Co; 1988: chap 81, with permission.

documentation of injury. The Committee on Adolescence has published a sample "Sexual Assault Data Sheet" (Table 16). The AAP Committee on Child Abuse and Neglect in the statement on the Evaluation of Sexual Assault provides helpful information regarding specific situations encountered in the sexually assaulted child or adolescent. These include the need for cultures, indications for pregnancy, prophylaxis (Table 16). Recommendations for the treatment or prophylaxis of sexually transmitted disease in children may be obtained either from the *Red Book* published by the AAP Committee on Infectious Disease or "Sexually Transmitted Diseases Treatment Guidelines" published in *Morbidity and Mortality Weekly* by the CDC.

Suicide and Psychiatric Emergencies

Suicide and psychiatric emergencies are crisis situations for both the child and the family. "Cluster suicide" has also emerged in recent years to describe the occurrence of multiple suicides during a short period of time in the same geographic location. To respond effectively to these types of suicide or psychiatric crises, physicians and EDs must have developed working relationships with colleagues in the community in child psychiatry and clinical psychology, local mental health agencies, family and children's services, crisis hot lines, and crisis intervention centers. One of these agencies may be of assistance in managing the case described earlier of the disturbed adolescent who locked herself in the bathroom. There must be a mechanism in place for immediate psychiatric consultation and inpatient hospitalization or referral. In addition, the physician should become familiar with state and national sources that are concerned with youth suicide and local laws pertaining to involuntary commitment. The social services department can help in preparing a list of these resources and their telephone numbers. The list should be kept posted in the ED or office setting and updated annually.

Table 16. — Sample Sexual Assault Data Sheet*

I. History

    A. Presentation in Emergency Department

        1.   Date seen _____

        2.   Time seen _____ am _____ pm

        3.   Mode of entry: police _____ friend _____

                        family _____ self-referral _____

                        other _____

    B. Date of assault _____

    C. Time of assault _____ am _____ pm

    D. Circumstances of assault (including postassault activity, changes of clothing, bathing, douching. Record evidence of torn clothing, bruises, blood, and semen stains):

_____

_____

_____

    E. Menarche _____

    F. Last menstrual period _____

    G. Method of birth control _____

    H. Current medications: Yes _____ No _____

II. Physical examination

    A. General appearance (include the emotional state, behavior of patient. Document areas of obvious trauma by photograph or diagram):

_____

_____

_____

    B. T _____ P _____ BP _____ Wt _____ Pubertal stage
       (Tanner)

_____

    C. Evidence of trauma:

_____

_____

Table 16. — Sample Sexual Assault Data Sheet* (continued)

D. Description of clothing:
    _____ torn
    _____ blood-stained
    _____ semen-stained
    _____ normal

E. Description of perineum:
    _____ normal
    _____ laceration
    _____ ecchymosis
    _____ bleeding

F. Pelvic examination:
    _____ vagina
    _____ cervix
    _____ uterus
    _____ adnexa
    _____ rectum

III. Laboratory evaluation

Results	Done	Not Done	
A. Wet preparation of vaginal fluid for motile sperm and *Trichomonas vaginalis*	_____	_____	_____
B. Vaginal washing for			
1. Acid phosphatase	_____	_____	_____
2. ABH agglutinogen	_____	_____	_____
C. Culture of vagina for *Neisseria gonorrhoeae* (GC)	_____	_____	_____
D. Culture of anus for GC	_____	_____	_____
E. Culture of oropharynx for GC	_____	_____	_____
F. Culture of urethra for GC	_____	_____	_____
G. Serologic test for syphilis	_____	_____	_____
H. Pregnancy test (pubertal females)	_____	_____	_____
I. Wood's lamp for semen	_____	_____	_____
J. Hair combing of pubis	_____	_____	_____
K. Fingernail scrapings			
L. Serum sample frozen and saved for future testing	_____	_____	_____
M. *Chlamydia* culture (where available)	_____	_____	_____

IV. Therapy (if indicated)   Dose given
   A. Antibiotic prophylaxis (in accordance
      with current Centers for Disease
      Control recommendations for areas
      of antimicrobial resistant gonococcal
      strains):
      Ceftriaxone, 250 mg, IM
      PLUS
      Doxycycline, 100 mg, by mouth,
      twice a day for 7 days
      OR   _____
      Tetracycline HCL, 500 mg, by mouth,
      4 times a day for 7 days.
      Tetracycline should not be given to
      patients who are pregnant or to those
      allergic to tetracycline. In areas
      where resistant strains of N gonorrhoeae
      are nonendemic, regimens known to be less
      effective against antibiotic-resistant
      strains may be used.   _____
   B. Tetanus toxoid as indicated according to
      Public Health Service recommendations   _____
   C. Pregnancy prevention for females[†]
      Ethinyl estradiol 5 mg/d x 5 days, or Ovral,
      2 mg (1 tablet) every 3 hours x 4, or 2 tablets
      in 2 divided doses 6 hours apart   _____

V. Reported to police: Date _____ Time _____

VI. Disposition and follow up: _____
   _____
   _____

*From American Academy of Pediatrics, Committee on Adolescence. Rape and the adolescent. *Pediatrics.* 1988;81:595-597, with permission.

†The use of pregnancy prevention drugs in females who have been raped is controversial. First, nausea and vomiting secondary to estrogens are common and warrant vigorous counseling at the time of prescription. Such symptoms can be especially unpleasant given the circumstances and can lead to noncompliance. Second, such drugs are associated with a small failure rate. Third, their teratogenic potential is not entirely clear. Finally, the incidence of pregnancy after rape is extremely low, lower than predicted from random single acts of intercourse, so the wisdom of using these drugs is questionable. The practitioner who chooses to use those drugs should be fully informed about these factors and should share these facts with the patient.

Written policies and procedures should cover identification of high-risk patients, indications for hospitalization, notification of ancillary personnel such as security and social services, and the use of medication and restraints. High-risk situations for suicide include suicide attempt just made, suicidal threat made, "accidental" ingestion, complaints of depression, appearance of depression, aggressive violent behavior, psychotic child, significant withdrawal by the child, perceived or actual serious school problems, family stress, or peer pressures. The need for hospitalization or immediate referral following a suicide attempt or gesture must also be determined. Many psychiatrists believe that all children who have made a suicide attempt or gesture or who have exhibited attention-seeking behavior that may be suicidal should be hospitalized. If controversy or doubt exists, the need for hospitalization should be determined on the basis of an evaluation of the social situation, perceived intent of the victim, potential lethality of method, history, precipitating events, current mental status, and support of family, peers, and teachers.

The protocol developed for the physician evaluation of the suicidal or psychiatric patient must attend to the assessment and care of both the child and the family. The physical condition of the child must be determined during the emergency assessment, with special attention to diagnosing medical conditions or intoxications that mimic psychiatric emergencies. On the other hand, psychiatrically impaired children may also have coexisting medical problems that require immediate attention.

Poisoning—Poison Control Centers

Because of the frequency and variety of toxicologic emergencies in children, the primary care physician must be part of or have access to a regional poison control network. A list of Regional Poison Control Centers is provided in Appendix N. Through the network the facility must have immediate access to poison control information and acute care protocols and must be prepared to provide suitable psychiatric consultation or referral. The network should be able to respond to telephone referrals/consultations and provide immediate information concerning therapy or referral to a regional poison information center. The ED must also maintain some on-site resources. These would include protocols for common pediatric ingestions, a readily available reference chart of antidotes, the availability of laboratory tests, medications, an equipment list, and a reference library.

Sudden Infant Death Syndrome

Cases of sudden infant death syndrome (SIDS) require a great deal of sensitivity and clinical expertise on the part of the physician and ED staff. With the infant's death, the family is in a state of crisis. While going through this emotionally difficult period, family members must cope with the investigation into the infant's death and subsequent need for autopsy. An organized approach will help to ensure that both a thorough diagnostic study is done and the family's needs are addressed.

Since SIDS is a diagnosis of exclusion, the differential diagnosis must be carefully considered at the time of the infant's death. Especially important is the fact that homicide is the leading cause of injury mortality in children under 1 year of age. Homicide, child abuse, or child neglect fatalities may be misdiagnosed or incorrectly reported as SIDS. There are a number of "red flags" to alert the physician to the need for a more intensive investigation (Table 17). Environmental or infectious causes must also be considered, especially when there is a history of lethargy or vomiting prior to death. Toxicologic studies should be conducted when there is a history of substance abuse among family members or when there is a suggestion of drug or substance abuse present at the scene. All cases of SIDS should be referred to the medical examiner. All cases

Table 17. — Historical Items Necessitating Further Investigation of Sudden Infant Death

History of severe depression or mental illness of the caretaker

More than one unexplained infant death in the family

A prior history of child abuse or neglect of the deceased infant or a sibling

Prior unexplained collapses of the infant necessitating emergency treatment

Prolonged period between the collapse and the notification of emergency personnel

---

should be referred to the police to address the need for a death scene investigation. The family should be given immediate support through the hospital chaplaincy or social services. The telephone numbers or information concerning local organizations such as Compassionate Friends should be kept readily available to provide to the family for future support or, alternatively, the ED may contact the group to refer the family. A listing of SIDS Centers is provided in Appendix O. Additional consideration should be given, when deemed appropriate, to scheduling a postmortem conference with the family. At this time the family may be offered additional support and be provided with the results of the infant's postmortem examination. Generally this visit should be scheduled within a month of the infant's death.

Deaths in the Emergency Department

The death of a child is always a traumatic and difficult experience. The grief of parents and family may be overwhelming. As in the scenario depicted, when contacted about sudden unexpected death of one of your patients, you, the primary care provider, may have significant impact on both the surviving family members as well as on the ED staff. In advance of any pediatric deaths, it would be appropriate for the physician to review the policies and procedures in existence for death of a child in an emergency situation (Table 18). Some institutions have found a checklist that outlines actions and procedures in the event of a child's death useful (Table 19). The ED must have an area where the parents and family of a child who is critically ill or has died may grieve in private. For the child who has arrived gravely ill or injured or who is dead on arrival, staff contact with the family must be established quickly and maintained. When the parents are informed of the child's death they should be given the opportunity to hold or be with the child. Many parents will need time to decide how they feel. Parents should always be offered help from the hospital chaplaincy or social services and assistance in contacting relatives, friends, or clergy.

Following a period during which the parents have been allowed to be with the child or grieve in private, they should be informed of the need for autopsy and what the state laws are concerning mandatory request for organ donation. In all but select circumstances, autopsies should be requested regardless of legal requirements. In most cases of deaths that occur in the ED, only the cornea will be suitable for organ donation.

Many quality assurance programs for the ED contain provisions for a monitoring of all deaths that occur in the ED or within 48 hours of admission from the ED. Under most circumstances deaths that occur in the ED will be referred to the medical examiner for evaluation. Physicians should be familiar with their local and state laws concerning the need for postmortem examination. Generally, the case should be referred to the medical examiner if no physician was in attendance at the time of death or if the death was sudden, violent, suspicious, or not the result of natural causes. In many jurisdictions the medical examiner will request that all tubes and lines that were in place at the time of death be left in position. The physician needs to document clearly in the medical record the circumstances, physical examination, and time of death.

Table 18. — Sample Hospital Protocol for Child Fatalities

This protocol represents the minimum criteria to be performed on all child deaths (0-15 years) that occur in the Emergency Department (ED) or in the inpatient setting in a hospital within 24 hours of the time of admission. A uniform report form documenting completion of the protocol must be completed before the child's body can be released.

The coroner/medical examiner should be notified by the ED physician or nursing supervisor (or equivalent role) for:

All ED deaths

All dead-on-arrival cases

All deaths in the inpatient setting of a hospital that occur within 24 hours of admission.

A social service consultation should be seriously considered to provide family support and an assessment of family needs/concerns.

Complete a medical record including the history of the circumstances leading to the child's death, mechanism of injury, events leading to the child's death, and supervision at time of death or injury. Notation should be made as to the source of the above information. The physical examination should include, at a minimum, the child's weight, height, head circumference if 1 year of age or under, core body temperature (rectal), and documentation of the examination of the fundi, skin to include assessment of ecchymosis, burns, lacerations and other defects of the skin, lividity and rigidity, and genitalia. The medical record should also include the time of death and physician who pronounced the child dead.

For deaths occurring within 24 hours of admission, a death note shall be entered into the medical record by the physician in attendance at the time of the child's death and will include nature of the presenting injury/illness.

If instructed by the coroner/medical examiner, all clothing and personal effects should be bundled, secured under lock, and a "chain of custody" form initiated.

All tubes and lines should be left in place after the child's death.

For children 1 year of age or under, when the cause of death is undetermined or sudden infant death syndrome is suspected, a skeletal survey should be obtained to include separate anteroposterior and lateral views of the skull, extremities, chest, abdomen, pelvis, and spine.

If possible, the child's body should be stored under refrigeration unless taken directly to the medical examiner.

Table 19. — Checklist for Cases Involving Children Who Die or Are Dead on Arrival in the Emergency Department

_____ 1. Notification of coroner/medical examiner. Instructions taken for disposition of clothing/personal effects.

_____ 2. Discuss request for autopsy with family and medical examiner in all cases.

_____ 3. Notification of law enforcement (or ensure coroner/medical examiner has notified law enforcement) if:
   • Sudden infant death syndrome
   • Abuse
   • Undetermined cause of death
   • Other instances of suspected homicide or suicide

_____ 4. Notification of Division of Family Services if abuse/neglect by an adult who has care, custody, or control of the child.

_____ 5. Medical record completed and contains:

   Name
   Birth date
   History of circumstances of illness or injury leading to child's death, source of information
   Weight
   Height
   Core body temperature (rectal)
   Head circumference if 1 year of age or under
   Description of fundi; skin to include assessment of ecchymosis, burns, lacerations, rigidity, lividity; genitalia
   Time of death
   Signature of physician of record
   Death note

_____ 6. Social service consultation, including name of social service professional.

_____ 7. Request for organ donation, after notice to coroner/medical examiner.

_____ 8. Need for skeletal survey, or other appropriate laboratory tests.

There should be a request for an autopsy. The medical examiner is under no obligation to perform one unless homicide is to be ruled out. In some jurisdictions all children in whom sudden infant death syndrome is suspected are autopsied. In other cases, if the family is not asked and the medical examiner decides not to do a postmortem, then the opportunity is lost.

The physical examination in cases of death in the ED should include a statement that the patient was apneic, pulseless, with no motor activity, and the pupils were fixed and dilated. If the possibility of homicide or suicide exists, the police will need to be notified. The patient's clothing needs to be bundled and either kept for the coroner or police or in other circumstances given to the family.

The needs of ED staff members must also be addressed. Although the professionals in the ED may have experienced the death of a child on previous occasions, circumstances may dictate a recovery time period for those who have been directly involved and/or a postmortem conference to allow staff to express their feelings and evaluate the team's performance.

Conclusions

The primary care provider is critical in planning that the needs of children are met during special situations in emergency medical services. That involvement includes checking to see that protocols with pediatric components exist, helping to establish new or revised protocols, and serving either directly or as a resource in the care of these children.

Mass Casualty/Disaster Planning
JCAHO Manual

Action Points

1. Of the emergency facilities that you use, review their existing guidelines for mass casualties, unaccompanied minors, child abuse, psychiatric emergencies (including poisoning and suicidal ideation), and deaths in the ED. If existing documents are found insufficient for the care of your patients, offer assistance in rewriting these policies and procedures.

2. Be involved and familiar with local disaster plans.

3. Determine your role in the care of pediatric patients who are victims of a mass casualty.

4. Should they not exist, prepare office guidelines for the care of unaccompanied minors.

5. Know how to access the local child abuse agency and be familiar with your state's statutes regarding child abuse.

6. Explore the availability of your community's mental health agencies, crisis hot lines, and crisis intervention centers.

7. Assume responsibility for counseling bereaved family members, conducting a follow-up death conference, and making appropriate referrals, especially for a family who has experienced a sudden unexpected death in the ED.

8. Be familiar with local and state laws regarding the need for postmortem exami- nations.

AAP Resources

American Academy of Pediatrics, Committee on Infectious Diseases. *Report of the Committee on Infectious Diseases*, 1991. 22nd ed. Elk Grove Village, IL: American Academy of Pediatrics, 1991

Bibliography

Unaccompanied Minor

Holder AR. Minors' rights to consent to medical care. *JAMA*. 1987;257:3400-3402

Neinstein LS. Consent and confidentiality laws for minors in the western United States. *West J Med*. 1987;147:218-224

Selbst SM. Treating minors without their parents. *Pediatr Emerg Care*. 1985;1:168-173

Child Abuse and Sexual Assault

American Academy of Pediatrics, Committee on Adolescence. Rape and the Adolescent. *Pediatrics*. 1988;81:595-597

American Academy of Pediatrics, Committee on Adolescence. Role of the pediatrician in management of sexually transmitted diseases in children and adolescents. *Pediatrics*. 1987;79: 454-456

American Academy of Pediatrics, Committee on Child Abuse and Neglect. Guidelines for the evaluation of sexual abuse of children. *Pediatrics*. 1991;87:254-260

American Academy of Pediatrics, Committee on Child Abuse and Neglect. Public disclosure of private information about victims of abuse. *Pediatrics*. 1991;87:261

Ludwig S. Child abuse. In: Fleisher GR, Ludwig S, eds. *Textbook of Pediatric Emergency Medicine*. 2nd ed. Baltimore, MD: Williams & Wilkins Co; 1988: chap 81

1989 Sexually transmitted diseases treatment guidelines. *MMWR*. 1989;38(suppl 8):1-43

Suicide and Psychiatric Emergencies

American Academy of Pediatrics, Committee on Adolescence. Suicide and suicide attempts in adolescents and young adults. *Pediatrics*. 1988;81:322-324

Poisoning—Poison Control Centers

Litovitz TL, Schmitz BF, Bailey KM. 1989 Annual Report of the American Association of Poison Control Centers National Data Collection System. *Am J Emerg Med*. 1990;8:394-442

CHAPTER 10

ADVOCATING FOR EMS-C ON A BROADER SCALE

Case

A preadolescent girl sustains multiple injuries in a fall from her garage roof. Her condition was initially stabilized at a local hospital and she was then transferred at your request to the care of a pediatric surgeon at a tertiary care center. The child was placed in the intensive care unit. The child's mother calls your office the morning following admission to discuss her child's progress.

Questions

1. What roles does the primary care provider play in the multiple disciplinary system of Emergency Medical Services for Children (EMS-C)?

2. After eventual stabilization, what responsibilities exist for the primary care provider who may not remain intimately involved with management decisions for the critically ill or injured child?

Key Term

Medical Home: Under this concept medical care should be accessible, continuous, comprehensive, family centered, coordinated, and compassionate. For full recommendations regarding medical home, see AAP Policy "The Medical Home" (Appendix P).

The Role of the Primary Care Provider

The majority of primary care providers already play an active role in EMS-C. As the "medical home" for the child and family, they offer continuity of care that is comprehensive and accessible. With periodic child health supervision visits, they are the primary focus for prevention and early intervention programs. Immunizations offer illness prevention; discussions and education on safety such as car restraint devices and bicycle helmets alert the family and child to potential injury. Hopefully the primary care provider has alerted and instructed the family on how to access the community's EMS-C system as part of anticipatory guidance. First aid and emergency care with awareness of the 911 system and the transport team is of utmost importance.

In all circumstances, primary care providers remain advocates for the child and family. Primary care providers practice child advocacy when they maintain close liaison with family, the emergency department (ED), and hospital, especially at times of acute illness and injury. In the case scenario presented above, the primary care provider will assist the child and family by assuring communications between the original ED specialists and other subspecialists. Physicians will strengthen child advocacy if they support communication and continuity of care for their community's paraprofessionals; ED personnel; and intensive care, hospital, and rehabilitation specialists (Fig 3).

Advocacy is an ongoing process for the primary care provider. The physician may be actively involved in direct care with child health supervision and anticipatory guidance; in referral at the time of a crisis or emergency, acting in coordination with the intensivist and rehabilitation specialist; or in acting collectively in public advocacy (Fig 4).

In the local and state community organizations, public and private, there are many groups currently actively involved as advocates for injury prevention and improving immunization levels. The Junior Leagues, Kiwanis and Rotarians, Pop Warners, and Police Activities Leagues are examples of lay public groups interested in various facets of EMS-C system of advocacy. Public institutions such as the Health, Education, Human Services, and Transportation Departments offer other areas for promotion of education and preventive services for accidents, injuries, and illnesses. Health insurance groups

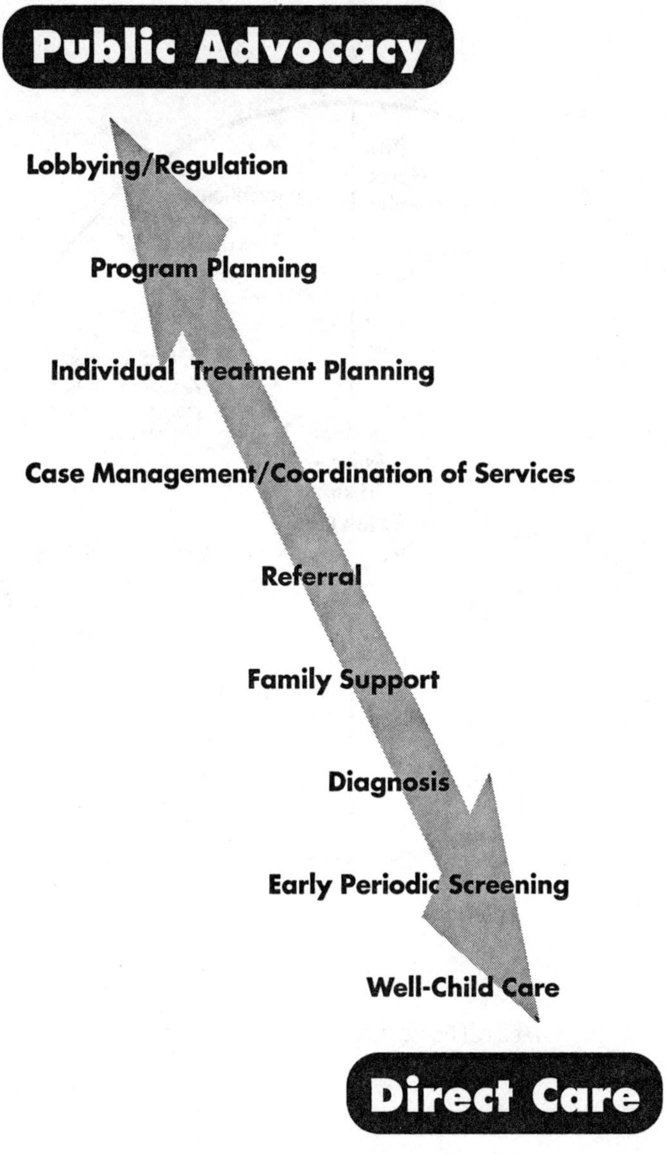

Public Advocacy

Lobbying/Regulation

Program Planning

Individual Treatment Planning

Case Management/Coordination of Services

Referral

Family Support

Diagnosis

Early Periodic Screening

Well-Child Care

Direct Care

Fig 3. Child Advocacy: Modes of Involvement.

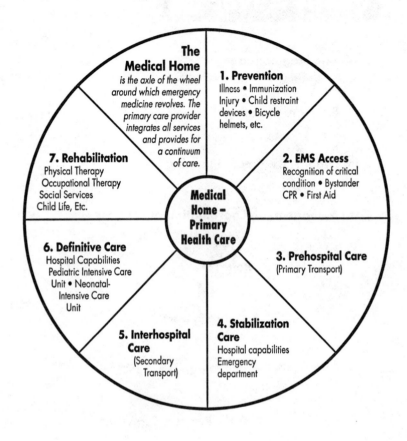

The
Medical Home
is the axle of the wheel
around which emergency
medicine revolves. The
primary care provider
integrates all services
and provides for
a continuum
of care.

1. Prevention
Illness • Immunization
Injury • Child restraint
devices • Bicycle
helmets, etc.

7. Rehabilitation
Physical Therapy
Occupational Therapy
Social Services
Child Life, Etc.

Medical Home – Primary Health Care

2. EMS Access
Recognition of critical
condition • Bystander
CPR • First Aid

6. Definitive Care
Hospital Capabilities
Pediatric Intensive Care
Unit • Neonatal-
Intensive Care
Unit

3. Prehospital Care
(Primary Transport)

5. Interhospital Care
(Secondary
Transport)

4. Stabilization Care
Hospital capabilities
Emergency
department

Fig 4. Medical home model of primary health care.

and hospitals are also vitally concerned with early access to emergency medical care and prevention. Nonprofit, professional associations such as the American Academy of Pediatrics and American College of Emergency Physicians are involved as advocates for injury prevention. The individual physician should work within the local community to stimulate organized efforts in advocacy for an effective EMS-C system.

Under the EMS-C demonstration grants through the Bureau of Maternal and Child Health, there are many practical applications for individuals or chapters to utilize. The Hawaii EMS-C grant under Wallace Matthews, MD, initiated an injury prevention program called "Kids in Sports." Under the same grant, Joseph Young, MD, led a project utilizing pediatricians to focus on safety and health education in the elementary school with "Adopt-a School" program. Robert Luten, MD, focused attention on the "Year of the Child in Emergency Medical Services" (now known as the Children's Emergency Medical Services Alliance), not only in his state of Florida but nationally. His advocacy group included supporting national organizations, hospitals, and pharmaceutical supply offices. *Emergency Medical Services for Children Innovation Bank*, March, 1991, third edition, contains many examples of advocacy within the EMS-C system. Single copies can be obtained from the National Maternal and Child Health Clearinghouse, Washington, DC.

Nationally, in late 1986, the Bureau of Maternal and Child Health and Resources Development of the US Department of Health and Human Services, with assistance from the Centers for Disease Control and the National Highway Traffic Safety Administration, established the National Committee for Injury Prevention and Control. The project was managed and staffed by Education Development Center, Inc of Newton, Massachusetts. *Injury Prevention: Meeting the Challenge*, by the National Committee and Education Development Center, is the result of that collaboration. This book is a must for all advocates involved in prevention of injuries.

It will help you organize your efforts and resources in making a meaningful approach to injury prevention as a community leader or advocate. Since unintentional and intentional injury to the body is of high priority in the AAP agenda, this book should be reviewed as you initiate your involvement in injury prevention.

In conclusion, advocacy begins with direct care of the patient. A comprehensive medical home model serves as the framework of this approach. Direct involvement at all levels in the care of the child enlarges the scope of services provided and establishes linkages that improve the health care for individual patients as well as for the community at large. Public advocacy on a local, county, state, or national level is essential to achieve a meaningful EMS-C system. Through these efforts better health care will be available to all of our children. Appendix Q shows an example of model legislation proposed in one state by an interested physician.

Action Points

1. Primary care physicians should work within their local communities to stimulate and foster organized efforts to create and sustain emergency medical systems for children.

2. Within their practices, primary care physicians should improve the linkage with all members of the emergency medical care system for children.

AAP Resources

American Academy of Pediatrics. *Government Affairs Handbook*. Elk Grove Village, IL: American Academy of Pediatrics; 1992

Federal Issues:
American Academy of Pediatrics, Department of Government Liaison. 1331 Pennsylvania Ave NW, Suite 721N, Washington, DC, 20004-1703, 202/662-7460

State Model Bills:
American Academy of Pediatrics, Division of State Government Affairs. 141 Northwest Point Blvd, Elk Grove Village, IL 60009-0927, 708/228-5005

Bibliography

Brewer EJ, McPherson J, Magrab PR, Hutchins VL. Family-centered community-based, coordinated care for children with special health care needs. *Pediatrics.* 1989;83:1055-1060

Narkewicz RM. Family-centered, community-based, coordinated care for children with special needs. *Pediatrics.* 1989; 83:1061

Sia CJ, Stewart JL. The medical home and PL 99-457 in Hawaii. *Hawaii Med J.* 1989;48:529-535

Sia CJ, Peter MI. Physician involvement strategies to promote the medical home. *Pediatrics.* 1990;85:128-130

Sia CJ, Breakey GF. The role of the medical home in child abuse prevention and positive child development. *Hawaii Med J.* 1985;44:242-247

APPENDIX A

AMERICAN ACADEMY OF PEDIATRICS

Provisional Committee on Pediatric Emergency Medicine

PEDIATRICIAN'S ROLE IN EMERGENCY MEDICAL SERVICES FOR CHILDREN (RE8115)

To reduce the morbidity and mortality of critically ill and injured children, comprehensive care must be provided. This includes effective services and treatment from the onset of the illness or injury through definitive care. Pediatricians should counsel families not only about prevention of disease and injury but also about access to pediatric emergency care resources in their region. If the interval between recognition of illness and delivery of care is to be reduced to a minimum, a prehospital protocol must be established. Parents as well as prehospital care providers must be knowledgeable about their community's prehospital protocol for life-threatening illness or injury.

Primary care pediatricians need to establish networks with hospital-based pediatricians, emergency physicians, pediatric surgeons, and other pediatric medical and pediatric surgical specialists so that there is clearly assigned responsibility for provision of pediatric emergency care.[1] When available, a pediatric emergency care delivery system will be comprehensive and designed to meet the unique needs of children. The specific objectives of an emergency medical services for children (EMS-C) system should remain constant even though available resources

*Reprinted with permission from American Academy of Pediatrics, Provisional Committee on Pediatric Emergency Medicine. Pediatrician's Role in Emergency Medical Services for Children. *Pediatrics.* 1988; 81:735.

may vary from region to region. For an EMS-C system to be most effective, practitioners need to develop the knowledge, skills, attitudes, and experience necessary to provide essential life support for ill and injured children.

Many regions currently have well-developed emergency medical services (EMS) systems with outstanding capability and sophistication but most have been designed to meet the needs of adults.[2] Pediatricians should advocate for modification of emergency delivery systems to include the components necessary for the special needs of the child. Such EMS-C systems should be responsible for both medical and surgical emergencies. Where population density is adequate, pediatricians should concentrate their referrals of critically ill and injured children to the EMS-C center to provide adequate patient volume for maintenance of skills and cost-effectiveness. Through a united effort, pediatricians should assure emergency department coverage on a 24-hour basis by physicians educated about, experienced in, and committed to the provision of optimum pediatric emergency care. Input and supervision by both pediatricians and other pediatric specialists are essential for the appropriate development, implementation, and monitoring of the ideal EMS-C system.

Provisional Committee on Pediatric Emergency Medicine (1986-1988)

Martha Bushore, MD, Chairperson
J. Alexander Haller, Jr, MD
Thomas Rice, MD
James S. Seidel, MD
Joseph E. Simon, MD
Calvin C. J. Sia, MD
Jonathan Singer, MD
F. Carden Johnston, MD

Liaisons

Gary Fleisher, MD
Max L. Ramenofsky, MD
Stephen Ludwig, MD
James O'Neill, MD
C. Randolph Turner, MD

References

1. Seidel JS: Emergency medical services and the pediatric patient: Are the needs being met? II. Training and equipping emergency medical services providers for pediatric emergencies. *Pediatrics.* 1986;78:808-812
2. Bushore M: Pediatric emergency care: Where do we go from here? A pediatrician's view. *Pediatr Emerg Care.* 1986;2:258-260

APPENDIX B

FEDERAL EMS-C GRANTS — CONTACT PERSONNEL

Alabama*
Randall Powell, MD
205/471-7994
FAX 205/471-7480

Alaska
Larry Bussone, MSW, MPA
907/465-3027
FAX 907/586-1877

Arkansas*
Debra Fiser, MD
501/320-1845
FAX 501/320-4264

California
Deborah P. Henderson, RN, MA
310/328-0720
FAX 310/328-0468

District of Columbia
Jane Ball, RN, DrPh
202/745-5188
202/745-3356

Florida
Treesa Soud, RN
904/737-1799
FAX 904/549-4508

Hawaii*
Donna Maiava
808/735-5267
FAX 808/735-2151

Idaho
Paul Anderson
208/334-6611
FAX 208/334-5998

Louisiana*
Liz Berzas
504/587-7402
FAX 504/584-1838

Maine*
Patrick Cote, RN, EMT-P
207/622-7566
FAX 207/622-3616

Maryland*
Ameen Ramzy, MD
410/328-5074
FAX 301/328-4768

Michigan
Mirtha Beadle
517/335-8571
FAX 517/335-8582

Missouri
Steve Hise
314/751-6356
FAX 314/751-6010

Nevada
Sheryl I. Yount
702/687-3065
FAX 702/687-5751

New Hampshire
Janet Houston
603/650-1813
FAX 603/650-1493

New Jersey
Sally Mathews, MSEMT
609/292-6789
FAX 609/292-3580

New Mexico
Lenora Olson, MA
505/272-5066
FAX 505/272-6503

New York City
Marsha Treiber, MPS
212/561-3161
FAX 212/561-3001

New York State
Elise van der Jagt, MD
716/275-8138
FAX 716/275-8706

North Carolina
Manjoo Mittal, PhD
919/966-7627
FAX 919/966-6164

Ohio
Jane Heffernan, RN, MS
614/466-8932
FAX 614/644-9850

Oklahoma
Ken Cadaret
405/271-4408
FAX 405/271-8709

Oregon*
Cynthia Cristofani, MD
503/280-3632
FAX 503/280-3836

Texas
Pauline Van Meurs
512/458-7550
FAX 512/458-7407

Utah
Jan M. Buttrey
801/538-6722
FAX 801/538-6387

Vermont
Patrick Malone
802/863-7310
FAX 802/863-7577

Washington*
Dena Brownstein, MD
206/526-2599
FAX 206/527-3945

Wisconsin*
Nicky Anders
608/266-0737
FAX 608/267-4853

*Funding has expired but information about project activities is still available.

APPENDIX C

FEDERAL EMS-C GRANTS — GRANT PRODUCTS

EDUCATION AND TRAINING PROGRAMS

	AL	AK	AR	CA	DC	FL	HI	ID	LA	ME	MD	NM	NY	NC	OH	OR	UT	VT	WA	WI
Prehospital	✓	✓	✓	✓	✓	✓	✓	✓	✓	✓	✓	✓	✓			✓		✓	✓	✓
Nurse/Physician	✓		✓	✓	✓	✓	✓	✓	✓	✓	✓	✓							✓	✓
Pediatric Intubation			✓	✓	✓	✓	✓	✓	✓	✓						✓			✓	✓
Injury Prevention	✓		✓	✓	✓	✓	✓	✓	✓	✓	✓	✓				✓		✓		✓
EMS Access/911			✓		✓	✓	✓	✓	✓	✓	✓					✓	✓			
Intraosseous Infusion					✓	✓	✓	✓	✓	✓	✓	✓				✓				
First Aid/Home Care	✓							✓	✓	✓		✓				✓				
Video/IVD/Computer Programs			✓					✓	✓	✓							✓	✓	✓	

	AL	AK	AR	CA	DC	FL	HI	ID	LA	ME	MD	NM	NY	NC	OH	OR	UT	VT	WA	WI
Rural Education				✓					✓	✓		✓							✓	

STANDARD AND PROTOCOL DEVELOPMENT

	AL	AK	AR	CA	DC	FL	HI	ID	LA	ME	MD	NM	NY	NC	OH	OR	UT	VT	WA	WI
Prehospital Equipment			✓	✓	✓	✓	✓	✓	✓	✓	✓				✓	✓		✓	✓	✓
Prehospital Treatment/ Triage			✓	✓	✓	✓	✓	✓	✓	✓	✓	✓			✓	✓		✓	✓	✓
Intraosseous Infusion	✓			✓	✓	✓	✓	✓	✓	✓					✓	✓	✓	✓		
Hospitals				✓	✓			✓	✓	✓		✓			✓	✓		✓	✓	✓
Ambulatory Care Centers/Clinics			✓	✓																

DATABASES AND RESEARCH PROJECTS

	AL	AK	AR	CA	DC	FL	HI	ID	LA	ME	MD	NM	NY	NC	OH	OR	UT	VT	WA	WI
Scoring/Triage	✓	✓	✓	✓	✓	✓	✓	✓	✓	✓	✓	✓	✓		✓	✓		✓	✓	
Prehospital/ Emergency Department	✓	✓	✓	✓	✓	✓	✓	✓	✓	✓	✓	✓	✓	✓	✓	✓	✓	✓	✓	✓

	AL	AK	AR	CA	DC	FL	HI	ID	LA	ME	MD	NM	NY	NC	OH	OR	UT	VT	WA	WI
Pediatric Critical Care		✓		✓									✓			✓		✓		✓
Head/Spinal Cord Injury					✓	✓	✓		✓										✓	
Transport/Transfer	✓		✓					✓		✓	✓	✓	✓	✓			✓			
Child Abuse	✓					✓		✓				✓								✓

OTHER SYSTEM COMPONENTS

	AL	AK	AR	CA	DC	FL	HI	ID	LA	ME	MD	NM	NY	NC	OH	OR	UT	VT	WA	WI
Coalition Development				✓	✓	✓	✓	✓		✓					✓			✓	✓	
Quality Assurance				✓	✓	✓	✓	✓		✓	✓	✓				✓				
Rehabilitation/ Discharge Planning	✓	✓	✓	✓		✓					✓	✓				✓				
Legal Issues												✓								

	AL	AK	AR	CA	DC	FL	HI	ID	LA	ME	MD	NM	NY	NC	OH	OR	UT	VT	WA	WI
Interhospital FAX							✓													
Newsletters				✓			✓													

SPECIAL POPULATIONS

	AL	AK	AR	CA	DC	FL	HI	ID	LA	ME	MD	NM	NY	NC	OH	OR	UT	VT	WA	WI
Farm Families															✓				✓	
Handicapped/ Chronically Ill												✓				✓			✓	
Minority Access												✓					✓	✓		✓

In Addition to the Products Listed Above . . .

Emergency Medical Services for Children: A Report to the Nation describes the "state of the art" in EMSC. This 165 page book was written by EMSC working groups and is available at no cost from the National Center for Education in Maternal and Child Health. Call Pam Mangu at (703) 524-7802.

APPENDIX D

GLOSSARY OF EMS-C TERMS

Key Terms

Advanced Life Support (ALS): In addition to BLS capacity, this responder to an emergency can provide resuscitation drugs.

Advanced Pediatric Life Support (APLS): A course developed conjointly by the American Academy of Pediatrics and the American College of Emergency Physicians designed to provide a core of knowledge in pediatric emergency medicine; the goal of the course is to provide the physician with information necessary to assess and manage critically ill or injured children during the first 30-60 minutes in the emergency department.

Basic Life Support (BLS): A responder to an emergency who has the capabilities to provide adequacy of airway, ventilation, and circulation.

Emergency: Any condition that requires immediate medical attention in the opinion of the patient, family, or whoever assumes responsibility of bringing the patient to the attention of the physician.

Emergency Department Approved for Pediatrics (EDAP): Defines a facility with an institutional and professional staff commitment to provide care for the ill or injured child.

Emergency Medical Service System (EMS): A group of organizations that collectively provide care to acutely ill or injured individuals.

Emergency Medical Service System for Children (EMS-C): Describes the broad-based effort to provide for the acutely ill or injured child as a target group.

Emergency Medical Technician-Basic (EMT): A prehospital care provider who has a total of 100-120 hours of education, of which 10 hours (on the average) are devoted to pediatric clinical and didactic instruction.

Emergency Medical Technician-Paramedic (EMT-P): Or paramedic, is a provider who has had 1,000 or more hours of instruction.

Emergent: A medical condition that requires immediate medical attention; delay may be harmful to the patient and the disorder is acute and potentially threatens life or function.

Enhanced 911: A telephone-based system in which activation provides a dispatcher information regarding location of all calls, enabling a link to emergency systems by persons unable to communicate the exact address and phone number of a call, including young children.

Interhospital Transport: Indicates the interfacility transportation of a patient from a referring institution to a receiving hospital.

Local Pediatric Center (LPC): A hospital with secondary or tertiary pediatric care capabilities.

Medical Home: Under this concept medical care should be accessible, continuous, comprehensive, family centered, coordinated, and compassionate.

911: A telephone system that provides direct access to an EMS system; activation triggers a coordinated and medically directed ambulance dispatch.

Pediatric Advanced Life Support (PALS): A course developed conjointly by the American Academy of Pediatrics and the American Heart Association with the expressed goal of providing up-to-date information on various aspects of advanced life support for infants and children; the course integrates knowledge and motor skills into a clinically useful discipline.

Pediatric Critical Care Center (PCC): A hospital with the complete spectrum of pediatric subspecialty services including services to handle cases of pediatric trauma.

Prehospital Transport: The transportation of the patient from the field (for example, home, physician's office) to the hospital.

Secondary Transport: Synonymous with interhospital transportation.

Transfer Agreement: An agreement that delineates the responsibilities of both the referring and referral hospitals.

True Emergency: Any condition clinically determined to require immediate medical care. Conditions that are a threat to the patient's health are sufficient to be considered true emergency; life and limb need not be threatened.

Urgent: A medical condition that requires attention within a few hours and will be of danger if not attended to within that time frame; disorder is acute but not necessarily severe.

APPENDIX E

AMERICAN MEDICAL ASSOCIATION COMMISSION ON EMERGENCY MEDICAL SERVICES

PEDIATRIC EMERGENCIES

An excerpt from "Guidelines for the Categorization of Hospital Emergency Capabilities."

Endorsed by the American Academy of Pediatrics

Preamble

The purpose of these guidelines for the classification of pediatric emergency services is (a) to allow any given community to identify the level of care available for the critically injured or ill pediatric patient, and (b) provide guidance to hospitals and EMS systems as to the resources necessary to provide optimal care to these children. This is a necessary step in the development of EMS systems that meet the needs of the pediatric patient.

These systems require (1) patient and parent recognition of when to access the system and knowledge of how to access the system; (2) prehospital care providers with appropriate expertise in the assessment and treatment of infants, children and adolescents; (3) regional networking of hospitals at varying levels of pediatric sophistication with transport systems to ensure that the critically ill or injured child is promptly identified, stabilized, and brought to the tertiary pediatric center; (4) primary and secondary centers that have the level of expertise to care

From "Guidelines for the Categorization of Hospital Emergency Capabilities," Chapter 7, Copyright 1989, American Medical Association. Used with permission.

for the bulk of pediatric patients; (5) the development of pediatric tertiary care facilities with pediatric subspecialist availability for the complex patients; (6) pediatric rehabilitation and long term care programs; and (7) audit and quality assurance programs to review the care rendered.

This document only addresses one part of a system, the classification of hospital capabilities. The systems implementation process involves a triphasic approach:

1. The identification of the capabilities of an institution by that institution which will provide information on its compliance with the guidelines.

2. Verification of a given hospital's compliance or noncompliance with the guidelines by outside, noninvolved individuals, the verification site review.

3. Designation of the hospital, a political governmental process by which a legally empowered agency designates the level of care a given hospital can provide, based on the above verification process.

This process should not be viewed as an isolated event, but always kept in the context of creating an appropriate and optimal system of pediatric care. Thus, these guidelines describe institutions with three different levels of pediatric sophistication. The Level III primary care hospital has minimal pediatric resources but has the ability to stabilize seriously ill and injured children before transport. The Level II hospital has significant pediatric resources but lacks comprehensive subspecialty expertise. The Level I hospital has comprehensive pediatric resources available to provide definitive care for the most complex problems.

Each institution has its own role to play in an EMS system. Public education and medically directed prehospital triage should direct critical pediatric patients to Level I or Level II facilities. The Level III hospital provides a vital service in stabilization and transfer in areas where

Level I and Level II facilities are not readily accessible so that prompt, life-saving care can be given prior to transport. The Level II center can provide definitive care for most patients, serving the needs of its catchment area and preventing the tertiary facility from being "flooded." The Level I center is a regional referral center providing primary as well as tertiary services to its own immediate catchment area and acting as a patient care, research, and educational resource for its region.

The exact interplay of these institutions will vary from state to state and region to region, as will available resources. In regions with limited pediatric resources, the concentration of specialists in a comprehensive center will be important to avoid the fragmentation and dilution of care to children. The Level I center outlined in these guidelines describes the requirements for such a comprehensive center capable of bringing pediatric medical and surgical expertise to the bedside of acutely ill or traumatized children. This comprehensive approach is important because of the multispecialty teams required to care for these complex patients.

Institutions may choose to develop expertise in certain areas and not others. In some areas such as large metropolitan communities, there may be adequate pediatric resources so that multiple centers will coexist. Alternatively, pediatric expertise may be divided so that different institutions elect to concentrate on specific missions, eg, pediatric traumatic or pediatric medical emergencies. In such settings these guidelines can be used to define the personnel, facilities, and equipment requirements necessary to meet the institution's mission. If a regional EMS system only defines, for example, the subset of capabilities for the traumatized child; the critically ill children, representing up to 80% of the patient pool requiring critical care, will be underserved. Great care must be exercised in the designation process to avoid neglecting the needs of major groups of pediatric patients.

Thus, it is important that these guidelines be utilized synergistically to ensure that pediatric trauma is an integral part of an overall system to provide care for traumatized patients while simultaneously an integrated approach to all pediatric patients exists within an overall EMS system. Where a comprehensive effort in meeting the needs of children has not been undertaken, these young patients are deprived of the benefits that an organized EMS system brings to adult patients. Where such an effort is made, the outcome for children can be significantly improved.

Each region will have its own unique characteristics with varying resources for pediatric care. The major factor that must be considered by all regions is the identifiable measure of the commitment. This commitment entails not just the determination that patients with severe trauma or life-threatening medical illness be triaged to the appropriate facility, but perhaps as importantly, this commitment should entail a constant effective integration of all the specialties dedicated to the improvement of care for children.

Classification: Pediatrics

Level I
An institution capable of providing comprehensive, specialized pediatric care to any acutely ill or injured child. Usually a children's hospital or a large general hospital with a pediatric division providing comprehensive subspecialty pediatric medical and surgical services.

Level II
A hospital with a pediatric service capable of caring for the majority of pediatric patients, but with limited pediatric critical care and subspecialty expertise.

Level III

A hospital with a functioning Emergency Department capable of evaluation, stabilization, and transfer of seriously ill and injured pediatric patients. Such facilities should have formalized transfer agreements to higher levels of pediatric care. They should provide a vital service in stabilization and transfer in areas where level I and level II facilities are not readily accessible.

Guidelines	Levels (E = essential; D = desirable)		
	I	II	III
I. Hospital organization All physician/staff members listed shall be either Board Certified or Board Eligible and actively seeking certification. This standard includes subspecialty Boards/Certificates where applicable. Each member of the institution's medical staff shall be credentialed by the facility for the appropriate specialty, including trauma care where applicable. More than one area of practice in the surgical specialties may be covered by one individual with appropriate training and experience.			
1. Department of Pediatrics	E	E	
Chairman	E	E	
Emergency Medicine[1]	E	D	
Critical Care	E	D	
Cardiology	E	D	
Neurology	E	D	
Pulmonology	E	D	
Allergy/Immunology	E	D	
Gastroenterology	E	D	

Guidelines	Levels (E = essential; D = desirable)		
	I	II	III
Hematology/Oncology	E	D	
Nephrology	E	D	
Endocrinology	E	D	
General Pediatrics	E	E	
Infectious Diseases	E	D	
2. Department of Surgery			
General Surgery		E	E
Pediatric Surgery	E	D	
Cardiac Surgery		D	
Pediatric Cardiac Surgery	E	D	
Neurologic Surgery		E	
Pediatric Neurologic Surgery	E	D	
Urologic Surgery		E	D
Pediatric Urologic Surgery	E	D	
Gynecologic Surgery	E	D	D
Orthopedic Surgery		E	D
Pediatric Orthopedic Surgery	E	D	
Plastic and Maxillofacial Surgery	E	D	
Oral Surgery	E	D	
Ophthalmologic Surgery		E	
Pediatric Ophthalmologic Surgery	E	D	
Pedodontics	E	D	
Otorhinolaryngology	E	E	
Thoracic Surgery		D	D
3. Department of Anesthesia	E	E	D
Pediatric Anesthesia	E	D	
4. Emergency Department	E^1	E	E
5. Pediatric Trauma Service	E	D	
6. Radiology Department	E	E	E
Pediatric Radiology	E	D	
7. Specialist Availability			
In-house 24 Hours per Day			
Emergency Medicine	E^2	E	E
Pediatric Intensive Care	E^3	D	

Guidelines	Levels (E = essential; D = desirable)		
	I	II	III
Pediatric Surgery	E[3]	D	
Anesthesia	E[4]	E[5]	
Neurologic Surgery	E[3]	D	
On Call and Promptly Available			
Cardiology		D	
Pediatric Cardiology	E	D	
Neurology		D	
Pediatric Neurology	E	D	
Pulmonology		D	
Pediatric Pulmonology	E	D	
Allergy/Immunology		D	
Pediatric Allergy/lmmunology	E	D	
Gastroenterology		D	
Pediatric Gastroenterology	E	D	
Hematology/Oncology		D	
Pediatric Hematology/Oncology	E	D	
Nephrology		D	
Pediatric Nephrology	E	D	
Endocrinology		D	
Pediatric Endocrinology	E	D	
General Pediatrics	E	E	D
Radiology		E	E
Pediatric Radiology	E	D	
Infectious Disease		D	
Pediatric Infectious Disease	E	D	
Family Medicine (or Pediatrics)			E
Anesthesia		E	D
Neurosurgery		E	
Pathology		E	D
Pediatric Pathology	E		
Physical Medicine and Rehabilitation	E	D	
Psychiatry		E	D
Pediatric Psychiatry	E	D	
Orthopedic Surgery		E	D
Pediatric Orthopedic Surgery	E	D	

Guidelines	Levels (E = essential; D = desirable)		
	I	II	III
Microsurgery	E	D	
Cardiac Surgery		D	
Pediatric Cardiac Surgery	E	D	
Gynecologic Surgery	E	D	
Otorhinolaryngolic Surgery	E	E	D
Plastic and Maxillofacial Surgery	E	D	
Oral Surgery	E	D	
Pedodontics	E	D	
Ophthalmologic Surgery		E	D
Pediatric Ophthalmologic Surgery	E	D	
Hand Surgery	E	D	
Urologic Surgery		E	D
Pediatric Urologic Surgery	E	D	
General Surgery		E	E
Vascular Surgery		D	
Thoracic Surgery		D	
8. Department of Nursing			
Director of Nursing	E	E	E
Manager, Pediatric Nursing	E	E	
Pediatric Head Nurse, General Pediatrics	E	E	
Pediatric Clinical Specialist: ED, OR, ICU, PACU	E	D	D
Pediatric Nurse Education	E	E	E
Trauma Nurse Coordinator	E^6	E^6	

II. Facilities/Resources/Capabilities
  1. Emergency Department
    A. Personnel

	I	II	III
1. Designated Physician Director	E^2	E	E
2. Physician with a commitment to the care of the critically ill or injured child present in ED 24 hours per day	E^2	E	E
3. Pediatric consultant readily available		E	E

Guidelines	Levels (E = essential; D = desirable)		
	I	II	III
4. Pediatric trauma team	E[6]	D	
Immediately Available			
a. Trauma team leader as designated by the chief of trauma service	E[7]		
b. 2 additional MD members of trauma team	E		
c. Neurologic Surgery	E[3]		
d. Emergency Nurses	E[8]		
e. Respiratory Therapist	E		
f. Laboratory Technician	E		
g. Radiology Technician	E		
h. Anesthesia	E[4]		
i. Orthopedics	E		
Promptly Available			
a. Licensed/certified clinical social worker, as a member of an interdisciplinary team, shall provide families with psychotherapeutic services, which may include, but are not limited to, crisis intervention, grief counseling, advocacy, etc.	E		
5. Nursing Staff			
a. Designated Pediatric Nursing Director	E	D	
b. Designated ED Nursing Director		E	D
c. Pediatric Clinical Nurse Specialists	E	D	
d. General Staff experienced in pediatric emergency nursing care	E	E[9]	E[9]
e. Staff Educator in Pediatrics	E	E	D

Guidelines	Levels (E = essential; D = desirable)		
	I	II	III
6. Dedicated Pediatric Emergency Area	E	D	
7. Designated resuscitation area equipped for the resuscitation and stabilization of neonatal, pediatric/adolescent patients and of adequate size to accommodate a full resuscitation team, including trauma	E	E	D
B. Equipment			
1. Communication equipment with EMS system	E	E	E
2. Airway control and ventilation equipment			
a. Laryngoscopes: sizes 0,1,2,3 straight and curved	E	E	E
b. Bag-valve mask resuscitators: infant, child, and adult	E	E	E
c. Endotracheal tubes cuffed and uncuffed: 2.5-9.0 (2.5-6.0 uncuffed)	E	E	E
d. Suction and appropriate size catheters, 5-12 fr, yankauer	E	E	E
e. Airways	E	E	E
f. Oxygen	E	E	E
g. Tracheostomy and thoracostomy trays with tracheostomy tubes: size 0-3; chest tubes: size 16-28	E	E	E
h. Thoracotomy tray	E	E	
3. Cardiopulmonary monitors with pediatric capability;	E	E	E
Monitors with at least two pressure capability	E	D	

Guidelines	Levels (E = essential; D = desirable)		
	I	II	III
4. Catheters for intravenous and intraarterial lines (3-8 fr, 16-24 gauge, intraosseous needles)	E	E	E
5. Monitor-defibrillator with pediatric paddles 0-400 watt/sec capability	E	E	E
6. Trays for venisection suturing, plastics	E	E	E
7. Pediatric splints, casts, traction including equipment for cervical spine stabilization	E	E	E
8. NG tubes: #10-36 fr, 3 and 5 fr feeding tubes	E	E	E
9. Foley catheters #8-14	E	E	E
10. Dialysis catheters: infant, pediatric and adult	E	E	E
11. Medications in pediatric concentrations	E	E	E
12. IV solutions with both microdrip and high volume infusion sets	E	E	E
13. Pediatric LP and subdural trays	E	E	E
14. Burr-hole/ICP monitor tray	E		
15. Blood pressure cuffs: premie, infant, child, adult, thigh	E	E	E
16. Doppler for blood pressure monitoring	E	E	E
17. Non-invasive blood pressure monitor	E	E	E
18. Pulse oximeter	E	E	E
19. MAST suits: adult, adolescent, child	E	E	E
20. Infusion pumps with fractional cc infusion capability	E	E	E
21. Pediatric scales for weight measurement	E	E	E

Guidelines	Levels (E = essential; D = desirable)		
	I	**II**	**III**
22. Temperature control devices for patient, IV fluids, and blood	E	E	E
23. Printed pediatric drug dosage reference material readily available	E	E	E
24. Thermometer with range 28°-42°C	E	E	E
25. OB tray	E	E	E
C. Support Services In-house 24 hours per day			
1. Laboratory with microcapability and blood gas analysis, blood bank capabilities	E	E	D
2. X-ray availability	E	E	D
3. Respiratory Therapy	E	E	D
D. On Call and Promptly Available			
1. Clinical social worker, as a member of an interdisciplinary team, shall provide families with psychotherapeutic services, which may include, but are not limited to, crisis intervention, grief counseling and advocacy, as well as physical and sexual abuse protocols	E	E	E
2. Pastoral Care	E	E	E
3. Child Life Therapist	E	D	
2. Intensive Care Unit			
A. Separate Pediatric Unit	E	D	
B. Designated Pediatric Medical Director	E	D	
C. Pediatric ICU physician present in hospital 24 hours per day	E[3]	D	
D. Designated Pediatric Nursing Unit Manager	E	D	

Guidelines	Levels (E = essential; D = desirable)		
	I	II	III
E. Pediatric Nurse Specialist	E	D	
F. Equipment			
1. Invasive monitoring venous, arterial	E	E	
2. Invasive monitoring capabilities: cardiac output, pulmonary artery, ICP monitoring	E	D	
3. Cardiopulmonary monitors with at least 3 pressures	E	E	
4. Capnography	E	D	
5. Pulse oximeter	E	E	
6. Noninvasive blood pressure monitoring	E	E	
7. Pacemaker capability, including temporary transvenous pacemaker	E		
8. Pediatric ventilators	E	E	
9. Airway control equipment as listed in ED	E	E	
10. Appropriate emergency surgical trays, ie, cutdown, thoracotomy, ventriculostomy	E	E	
11. Pulmonary function measuring devices	E	D	
3. Operating Room			
A. Readily available and adequately staffed 24 hours per day	E	E	D
B. Nursing Unit Manager	E	E	E
C. Scrub and circulating nurse readily available	E	E	D
D. Post Anesthesia Care Unit (may be PICU) staffed 24 hours per day	E	D	D
E. Equipment			
1. Cardiopulmonary bypass	E		
2. Operating microscope	E	D	

Guidelines	Levels (E = essential; D = desirable)		
	I	II	III
3. Thermal control for patient, room and blood	E	E	E
4. X-ray capability including C-arm	E	D	
5. Cardiopulmonary monitoring with	E	E	E
at least 3 pressures	E	D	
6. Endoscopes and bronchoscopes	E	E	
7. Carniotome	E	E	
8. Fracture table	E	E	D
9. Pediatric anesthesia equipment	E	E	D
10. Noninvasive blood pressure monitoring	E	E	D
11. Pulse oximeter	E	E	E
12. Cardiac output equipment	E	D	
13. Pediatric instruments and equipment	E	E	D
4. Clinical Laboratory			
Available 24 hours per day:	E	E	E
1. Chemistry	E	E	E
2. Hematology	E	E	E
3. Serology	E	E	D
4. Blood bank	E	E	E
5. Blood gases	E	E	E
6. Microbiology	E	E	D
7. Toxicology	E	E	D
8. Drug Levels	E	E	D
9. Micro capability	E	E	D
5. Hemodialysis Capability/Transfer Agreement	E	E	
6. Burn Unit Availability/ Transfer Agreement	E	E	E
7. Pediatric Medical/Surgical Units			
A. Separate pediatric unit	E	E	
B. Pediatric Unit Nursing Director	E	E	
C. Pediatric nurses in appropriate staffing	E	E	

Guidelines	Levels (E = essential; D = desirable)		
	I	II	III
D. Equipment			
1. Airway equipment as in ED	E	E	
2. Oxygen, air, and suction	E	E	
3. EKG monitor/defibrillator	E	E	
4. Standard pediatric IV solutions, drugs, and supplies	E	E	
8. Radiology			
A. Immediately Available			
1. Routines 24 hours per day	E	E	E
B. Promptly Available			
1. Angiography 24 hours per day	E	D	
2. Ultrasound 24 hours per day	E	D	
3. CT scan 24 hours per day	E	D	
4. Nuclear medicine	E	D	
5. MRI scan	D	D	
9. Rehabilitation Medicine/Transfer Agreement			
A. Medical Director	E	D	
B. Properly trained staff to provide comprehensive approach	E	D	
10. Acute Spinal Cord Injury Management Capability/Transfer Agreement	E	E	E
11. Helipad	E	E	E
12. Transport Protocols and Transfer Agreement for Critically Ill and Injured Pediatric Patients	E	E	E
13. Participation in Regional Interhospital Transfer Program, Including Transfer Agreements	E	E	E
14. Pharmacy Staffed by Licensed Pharmacist			
A. In-house 24 hours per day	E	D	
B. Promptly available		E	D
15. Organ Procurement Program and Agreement	E	E	E

Guidelines	Levels (E = essential; D = desirable)		
	I	II	III
III. Quality Assurance			
1. Structured program	E	E	E
2. Review of all pediatric deaths	E	E	E
3. Review of all incident reports	E	E	E
4. Multidisciplinary pediatric trauma and resuscitation conferences	E	E	E
5. Maintain pediatric trauma registry	E	D	
6. Participate in pediatric trauma registry	E	E	E
7. Pediatric Nursing Audit	E	E	E
8. Review of all ED 7-day readmits	E	E	E
9. ED physician audit of pediatric patients	E	E	E
10. Review of pediatric transports and pre-hospital care	E	E	E
11. Review of regional systems of pediatric care	E	E	E
12. Participate in medical direction of EMS systems	E	E	E
IV. Community Programs			
1. Consultations with physicians and referral institutions	E	E	E
2. Public Education	E	E	E
3. Continuing Education Program for professional staff	E	E	E
4. Prehospital Care Providers Education	E	D	D
5. Outreach program to referral institutions	E	D	
V. Research			
1. Pediatric Trauma	E	D	
2. Pediatric Critical Care	E	D	
3. Pediatric Emergency Medicine institutions	E	D	

NOTES: PEDIATRIC EMERGENCIES

1. Requirements may be met by a Pediatric Emergency Department in a Department of Pediatrics or by a recognized administrative component of Pediatric Emergency Medicine within a Department of Emergency Medicine.

2. This requirement may be fulfilled by a physician (1) who is board certified/board eligible in pediatrics or board certified/board prepared in emergency medicine and (2) who demonstrates his/her commitment by engaging in the exclusive practice of pediatric emergency medicine a minimum of 100 hours per month, or has an additional one year of training in pediatric emergency medicine.

3. When a resident or other physician is utilized to fulfill this requirement the chief of the respective specialty service shall designate residents at the appropriate level of training who can provide the indicated treatment. Staff specialist shall be physically present within 30 minutes.

4. Requirements may be fulfilled by an anesthesiology resident and/or CRNA designated by the Chief of Anesthesia as capable of assessing emergent situations in pediatric patients and providing any indicated treatment. Where no facility in a region can provide in-house anesthesia coverage, this requirement may be met by an attending level pediatric critical care or pediatric emergency medicine physician designated as above by the Chief of Anesthesia. A staff specialist in pediatric anesthesia must be available promptly within 30 minutes. (In Level II facilities a staff specialist in anesthesia must be available within 30 minutes.)

5. A physician capable of pediatric airway management must be present in the hospital 24 hours/day. This could be a pediatrician, emergency medicine physician, anesthesiologist or surgeon.

6. In institutions that do not provide an organized trauma service, these criteria do not apply.

7. A staff level surgical team leader must be in-house within 30 minutes if a surgical resident is fulfilling this requirement. The staff surgeon will assume the team leader role on arrival. In the interim, leadership of the trauma team must be defined clearly by pre-established protocols. Such protocols should ensure that an attending level physician is physically present during the initial resuscitation.

8. If the Emergency Department is not always staffed to provide an adequate number of trauma nurses, nurses in the hospital with special training in pediatric trauma must be on call as members of the trauma team. At least two nurses per shift must have completed a pediatric trauma nurse course. These nurses may come from a Pediatric Unit.

9. There must be one nurse on each shift who has extra competence in pediatrics as demonstrated by completing a comprehensive pediatric emergency nursing course.

APPENDIX F

PARENT INSTRUCTIONAL MATERIAL RESOURCES

American Academy of Pediatrics. Shelov SP, ed. *Caring for Your Baby and Young Child.* New York, NY: Bantam Books; 1991

American National Red Cross. *Standard First Aid and Personal Safety.* 2nd ed. Garden City, NY: Doubleday & Co; 1979

Benjamin B, Benjamin AF. *In Case of Emergency: What to Do Until the Doctor Arrives.* Garden City, NY: Doubleday & Co; 1965

Fontana VJ. *A Parent's Guide to Child Safety.* New York, NY: Thomas Y Crowell Co; 1973

Health and safety units. In: American Red Cross and American Academy of Pediatrics. *American Red Cross Child Care Course.* Washington, DC: American Red Cross; 1990

Kuehl G. *CPR - The Way to Save Lives: Cardiopulmonary Resuscitation.* University City, MO: JD Heade Co; 1984

Mosher C, Consumer Guide editors. *Emergency First Aid.* New York, NY: Beekman House; 1978

Schmitt BD. *Your Child's Health: The Parents' Guide to Symptoms, Emergencies, Common Illnesses, Behavior, and School Problems.* New York, NY: Bantam Books; 1991

Smith B, Stevens G. *The Emergency Book: You Can Save a Life.* New York, NY: Simon & Schuster; 1991

APPENDIX G

AAP LIFE SUPPORT PROGRAMS

Introduction

In recent years three new courses in Pediatric Life Support have been developed and sponsored by the American Academy of Pediatrics (AAP), the American Heart Association (AHA), and the American College of Emergency Medicine (ACEP). The new courses are:

Pediatric Advanced Life Support (PALS) — the Resuscitation Course

Advanced Pediatric Life Support (APLS) — the Emergency Care Course

Neonatal Resuscitation Program (NRP) — the Newborn Resuscitation Course

These courses are now being offered in addition to Basic Life Support "C" (BLS) and Pediatric Basic Life Support (PBLS).

By disseminating these courses, the sponsoring organizations believe that health care professionals, both in and out of hospitals, will acquire and reinforce the skills needed in caring for the critically ill or traumatized child. It is further believed that the result of this skill enhancement will be a reduction in residual morbidity and, hopefully, mortality.

The rapid sequence with which the courses have appeared and the similarity in titles have engendered some confusion among potential enrollees regarding course content. This statement, endorsed by all three organizations, outlines objectives for each of the courses, briefly summarizes curriculum, and describes the potential target audiences.

The suggested sequence for completion of the courses by health care providers is:

1. Basic Life Support - "C" (BLS) or Pediatric Basic Life Support (PBLS)
2. Pediatric Advanced Life Support (PALS)
3. Advanced Pediatric Life Support (APLS)
4. Neonatal Resuscitation Program (NRP)

Basic Life Support For Health Care Providers (Course C) (BLS)

The BLS course has been taught for a number of years to professional health care providers. A current BLS-"C" Course card will fulfill the prerequisite requirement for acceptance into the PALS course.

Objective

The 1-day BLS course teaches background information about normal and dysfunctional cardiovascular anatomy and physiology, the principles of prevention and recognition of acute cardiovascular disease, and the technical aspects, including performance skills, of cardiopulmonary resuscitation (CPR) and foreign-body airway obstruction management. There are three courses (A, B, and C), but only the more advanced "C" module is recommended for health care professionals. It includes material on both adult and pediatric management.

Curriculum

Through a series of lectures, demonstrations, and hands-on mannequin and costudent teaching, the student is instructed in and practices adult one-rescuer CPR, child two-rescuer CPR, and pediatric foreign body airway obstruction management.

Audience

This AHA-sponsored course is appropriate for physicians, nurses, emergency medical technicians, and other health care providers.

For Course Information and Materials

For courses in your geographic area, contact the local affiliate of the American Heart Association.

Pediatric Basic Life Support (PBLS)

A current PBLS course card will fulfill the prerequisite requirement for acceptance into the PALS course.

Objective

The goals of this 1-day course are to teach the prevention of hazards to which infants and children may be exposed and the basic rescue techniques, such as cardiopulmonary resuscitation (CPR) and maneuvers for relief of foreign-body airway obstruction.

Curriculum

The material is presented in a series of lectures, demonstrations, and hands-on mannequin practice. The topics covered include cardiac and pulmonary arrest, basic resuscitation, and prevention of injury from safety hazards, including foreign-body airway obstruction.

Audience

This course is recommended for literally every person who may have responsibility for the care of children—parents, siblings, teachers, pediatric office workers, day-care personnel, and babysitters. It is given through the auspices of AHA, AAP, local hospital groups, prehospital emergency services, and school systems. Analogous courses are sponsored by the American Red Cross. Professionals who advise child care workers may find that taking the course is helpful in strengthening the effectiveness of their counseling.

For Course Information and Materials

The PBLS course is regularly offered by the Academy at the Spring Session and/or the Annual Meeting. Information about upcoming AAP-sponsored courses can be obtained by calling 800/433-9016, ext 6798. For courses in your geographic area, contact the local affiliate of the American Heart Association.

Pediatric Advanced Life Support (PALS)

Objective

This 2-day course is a structured core curriculum on pediatric resuscitation. It has been developed to teach management during the early minutes after critical presentation of the neonate, infant, child, or adolescent who has suffered a severe, life-threatening medical crisis.

It provides the information needed for recognizing the child at risk of cardiopulmonary arrest, strategies for preventing cardiopulmonary arrest in pediatrics, and reinforcement of the cognitive and psychomotor skills necessary for resuscitating and stabilizing the infant or child in respiratory failure, shock, or cardiopulmonary arrest.

Prerequisites

A current BLS-"C" or PBLS card is a prerequisite for enrollment in the PALS course.

Curriculum

PBLS is reviewed. More sophisticated presentations and management processes are introduced through concise lectures and at small-group skill stations. These include evaluation of cardiorespiratory status, airway management including bag-mask ventilation and intubation, vascular access and fluid therapy, appropriate usage of resuscitation equipment and medications, a pragmatic approach to rhythm disturbances, and a concise summary of neonatal resuscitation.

Practical application of these skills and their usage in critical situations is brought into focus through simulated case presentations. This is a two-step process utilizing large group discussions called "integration sessions" followed by small group teaching stations. Practical skill achievements are examined, and a written test is given.

Audience and Faculty

The course is sponsored by the Academy and the AHA. It is recommended that it be taken by all hospital-based health professionals who work with children, all office or clinic-based practitioners and nurses whose duties bring them into contact with children, and those with advanced training who provide emergency care before the hospital.

Course graduates with training as emergency, pediatric, or surgical nurse or physician, and physician assistants or prehospital emergency medical technicians are eligible to take designated instructor courses in order to be approved as faculty.

For Course Information and Materials

A PALS course is regularly offered by the Academy at the Spring Session and/or the Annual Meeting. Information about upcoming AAP-sponsored courses can be obtained by calling 800/433-9016, ext 6798.

For information about courses in your geographic area, contact the local affiliate of the American Heart Association.

Advanced Pediatric Life Support (APLS)

Objective

This 2 1/2 day course provides a detailed survey on the evaluation and management of pediatric medical and surgical emergencies. The course content is primarily oriented toward emergency diagnosis and response.

Knowledge and practice of pediatric resuscitation during the early minutes are reviewed. This experience is incorporated into the care of specific illnesses and trauma for the period the patient is being stabilized in the Emergency Department.

Prerequisites

A prior PALS course is recommended but is not a prerequisite.

Curriculum

Carefully focused lectures are presented on the topics of respiratory distress/failure, airway management, cardiopulmonary arrest, cardiac dysfunction, shock trauma of the chest, abdomen, head and neck, and neonatal emergencies. The course format combines lectures with small group sessions for case presentations and hands-on experience.

Topics covered in the interactive case management sessions include cardiorespiratory emergencies, head trauma, surgical trauma, environmental emergencies such as drowning and hyperthermia, neonatal emergencies, toxins, the trauma of child abuse, and conditions associated with an altered level of consciousness, including severe infections and diabetic ketoacidosis. There also are small group participatory stations on understanding the radiology of the pediatric airway and multiple sessions on "code" management simulations.

Appropriate pediatric resuscitation methods are repeatedly reviewed, practiced, and integrated into management of the specific medical and surgical diagnostic problems. Major life support procedures are performed hands-on, including vascular access techniques, chest tube placement, and needle cricothyreotomy.

Audience and Faculty

The course is sponsored by the Academy and the ACEP. It should be taken by all physicians and other health professionals who are responsible for the management of acutely ill children.

Faculty includes emergency, surgical, pediatric, and critical care physicians who have established competence in the management of pediatric emergencies and who have assimilated the course material.

For Course Information and Materials

An APLS course is regularly offered by the Academy at the Annual Meeting. Information about upcoming AAP-sponsored courses can be obtained by calling 800/433-9016, ext 6798.

The *Advanced Pediatric Life Support* manual is available for purchase from:

AAP Publications Department
141 Northwest Point Blvd
PO Box 927
Elk Grove Village, IL 60009-0927

For information about other APLS courses, contact:

American College of Emergency Physicians
ACEP National Course Coordinator
PO Box 619911
Dallas, TX 75261-9911
214/550-0911

Neonatal Resuscitation Program

Objective

This course has been designed to teach an appropriate stepwise approach to resuscitation of the newborn infant in the critical few minutes during and immediately following delivery. The causes, prevention, and management of mild-to-severe neonatal asphyxia are carefully defined and reiterated, so that health professionals may develop optimal competence in resuscitation.

Curriculum

This course is primarily designed to be used as an ongoing self-instructional, self-paced program, with an instructor guiding learners individually through the lessons. It can also be conducted over a 2-day period or in a series of classes over a period of several weeks.

A comprehensive instructional textbook forms the basic educational component of the program. Materials presented include pathophysiology of asphyxia, initial steps in resuscitation, bag-mask ventilation, chest compressions, intubation, and appropriate usage of medication. Under the direction of an approved instructor, self-study is integrated with hands-on practice of skills on mannequins for development of familiarity with equipment and its utilization. Emphasis is placed on anticipation and preparedness. Case presentations, written and hands-on testing, and considerable reiteration are utilized to help students assimilate the material.

Audience and Faculty

The course is sponsored by the Academy and AHA. It is recommended that it be taken by all health professionals who might find themselves in a situation requiring resuscitation of a newborn infant. There are no prerequisite courses, though PBLS might be helpful.

The faculty, including neonatologists, nurses, and pediatricians, have established competence in neonatal resuscitation and have been trained to serve as national, regional, or hospital-based instructors.

For Course Information and Materials

The Neonatal Resuscitation Program is administered by the Academy. Information about the program of study and approved instructors can be obtained by calling 800/433-9016, ext 6797.

The NRP course materials can be purchased from:

AAP Publications
141 Northwest Point Blvd
PO Box 927
Elk Grove Village, IL 60009-0927

APPENDIX H

PEDIATRIC REFERENCE MATERIALS - GENERAL

Adams FH, Emmanouilides GC, Riemenschneider TA, eds. *Moss' Heart Disease in Infants, Children and Adolescents.* 4th ed. Baltimore, MD: Williams & Wilkins; 1983

American Academy of Pediatrics, Committee on Infectious Diseases. *Report of the Committee on Infectious Diseases.* 22nd ed. Elk Grove Village, IL: American Academy of Pediatrics; 1991

Behrman RE, ed. *Nelson Textbook of Pediatrics.* 14th ed. Philadelphia, PA: WB Saunders Co; 1992

Chadwick DL, Berkowitz CD, Kearns D, et al, eds. *Color Atlas of Child Sexual Abuse.* Chicago, IL: Year Book Medical Publishers; 1989

Fitzpatrick TB, Arndt KA, Clark WH, et al. *Dermatology in General Medicine: Textbook and Atlas.* 3rd ed. New York, NY: McGraw-Hill; 1987

Greene MGG, ed. *The Harriet Lane Handbook: A Manual for Pediatric House Officers.* St Louis, MO: Mosby-Year Book, Inc; 1991

Krugman S, Katz SL, Gershon AA, Wilfert CM, eds. *Infectious Diseases of Children.* 9th ed. St Louis, MO: Mosby-Year Book, Inc; 1992

Ludwig S, Kornberg AE, eds. *Child Abuse: A Medical Reference.* 2nd ed. New York, NY: Churchill Livingstone; 1992

Markell EK, Voge M, John DJ. *Medical Parasitology.* 6th ed. Philadelphia, PA: WB Saunders Co; 1986

Ogden JA. *Pocket Guide to Pediatric Fractures.* Baltimore, MD: Williams & Wilkins; 1987

Rudolph AM, Hoffman JIE, eds. *Pediatrics.* 18th ed. Norwalk, CT: Appleton & Lange; 1987

Silverman FN, ed. *Caffey's Pediatric X-ray Diagnosis: An Integrated Imaging Approach.* 8th ed. Chicago, IL: Year Book Medical Publishers; 1985

Weinberg S, Prose NS. *Color Atlas of Pediatric Dermatology.* 2nd ed. New York, NY: McGraw-Hill Information Services Co; 1990

Zitelli BJ, Davis HW, eds. *Atlas of Pediatric Physical Diagnosis.* St Louis, MO: CV Mosby; 1987

PEDIATRIC REFERENCE MATERIALS - EMERGENCY MEDICINE

Alpert JJ, Reece R, eds. Symposium on Pediatric emergencies. *Pediatr Clin North Am.* 1979;26:705-764

Baldwin GA, ed. *Handbook of Pediatric Emergencies.* Boston, MA: Little, Brown & Co; 1989

Barkin RM, Rosen P, eds. *Emergency Pediatrics: A Guide to Ambulatory Care.* 2nd ed. St Louis, MO: CV Mosby; 1986

Black JA, ed. *Paediatric Emergencies.* 2nd ed. London, England: Butterworths; 1987

Burkle FM, Wiebe RA, eds. Pediatric Emergencies. In: *Emergency Medicine Clinics of North America.* Philadelphia, PA: WB Saunders Co; 1991:9

Chameides L, ed. *Textbook of Pediatric Advanced Life Support.* Dallas, TX: American Heart Association; 1988

Cohen SA. *Pediatric Emergency Management: Guidelines for Rapid Diagnosis and Therapy.* New York, NY: Appleton-Century-Crofts; 1982

Crain EF, Gershel JC, eds. *A Clinical Manual of Emergency Pediatrics*. Norwalk, CT: Appleton-Century-Crofts; 1986

Dieckmann RA. *Pediatric Emergency Care Systems*. Baltimore, MD: Williams & Wilkins Co; 1992

Ehrlich FE, Heldrich FJ, Tepas JJ, eds. *Pediatric Emergency Medicine*. Rockville, MD: Aspen Publishers; 1987

Eichelberger MR, Stossel-Pratsch GL, eds. *Pediatric Emergencies Manual*. Baltimore, MD: University Park Press; 1984

Fleisher GR, Ludwig S, eds. *Textbook of Pediatric Emergency Medicine*. 2nd ed. Baltimore, MD: Williams & Wilkins; 1988

Grossman M, Dieckmann RA, eds. *Pediatric Emergency Medicine: A Clinician's Reference*. Philadelphia, PA: Lippincott; 1991

Haller JA: *Emergency Medical Services for Children: Report of the 97th Ross Conference on Pediatric Research*. Columbus, OH: Ross Laboratories; 1989

Hamilton JP, Jacobs A, Morton D: *Pediatric Trauma Management for Emergency Medical Services*. 2nd ed. National Association of State EMS Directors and the Council of State Governments; 1989

Ludwig S, ed. Pediatric emergencies. In: *Clinics in Emergency Medicine*. New York, NY: Churchill Livingstone; 1985: vol 7

Ludwig S, Selbst S. A child-oriented emergency medical services system. *Curr Probl Pediatr*. 1990;20:3

Luten RC, ed. Problems in pediatric emergency medicine. In: *Contemporary Issues in Emergency Medicine*. New York, NY: Churchill Livingstone; 1988

Marcus RE. *Trauma in Children*. Rockville, MD: Aspen Publishers; 1986

Mayer TA, ed. *Emergency Management of Pediatric Trauma.* Philadelphia, PA: WB Saunders Co; 1985

Pierog JE, Pierog LJ, eds. *Pediatric Critical Illness and Injury: Assessment and Care.* Rockville, MD: Aspen Systems, Corp; 1984

Reece RM, ed. *Manual of Emergency Pediatrics.* 4th ed. Philadelphia, PA: WB Saunders Co; 1992

Seidel JS, Henderson DP, eds. Prehospital care of pediatric emergencies: management guidelines. LA Pediatric Society-American Academy of Pediatrics; 1987

Selbst SM, Torrey SB, eds. *Pediatric Emergency Medicine for the House Officer.* Baltimore, MD: Williams & Wilkins; 1988

Silverman BK, ed. *Advanced Pediatric Life Support.* Elk Grove Village, IL: American Academy of Pediatrics; Dallas, TX: American College of Emergency Physicians; 1989

Swischuk LE: *Emergency Radiology of the Acutely Ill or Injured Child.* 2nd ed. Baltimore, MD: Williams & Wilkins; 1986

Zanga JR, ed. *Manual of Pediatric Emergencies.* New York, NY: Churchill Livingstone; 1987

APPENDIX I

A RAPID METHOD FOR ESTIMATING WEIGHT AND RESUSCITATION DRUG DOSAGES FROM LENGTH IN THE PEDIATRIC AGE GROUP

Drug dosages used during pediatric emergencies and resuscitation are often based on estimated body weight. The Broselow Tape, a tape measure that estimates weight and drug dosages for pediatric patients from their length, has been developed to facilitate proper dosing during emergencies. In our study, 937 children of known weight were measured with this tape. Weight estimates generated by the tape were found to be within 15% error for 79% of the children. The tape was found to be extremely accurate for children from 3.5 to 10 kg, and from 10 to 25 kg. Regression lines of estimated compared with actual weight for these children have slopes of 0.98 and 0.96, respectively, not significantly different from the ideal slope of 1.00 (P = 28 and 13). Accuracy was significantly decreased for measured children who weighed more than 25 kg. In a separate group of children (n = 53), the tape was shown to be more accurate than weight estimates made by residents and pediatric nurses (P<.0001). Use of the Broselow Tape is a simple, accurate method of estimating pediatric weights and drug doses and eliminates the need for memorization and calculation.

Introduction

Drug dosages and fluid therapy used for pediatric resuscitation vary and are based on the patient's body weight. In a crisis situation, health care personnel may be unable to weigh patients, and the weight is estimated. The estimated weight then is used to calculate drug dosages by referring

Reprinted with permission. Lubitz DS, Seidel JS, Chameides L, Luten RC, Zaritsky AL, Campbell FW: A rapid method for estimating weight and resuscitation drug dosages from length in the pediatric age group. *Ann Emerg Med* 1988;17:576-581.

to charts, cards, or memory for the appropriate dose per kilogram of body weight.

Most methods currently used to estimate body weight in children are based on age.[1,2] Recently, several methods have been developed to estimate body weight based on height[3,4] and James Broselow has developed a simplified method of rapidly estimating weight based on height.[5]

In 1979, the National Center for Health Statistics (NCHS) published a new set of percentile curves for assessing the physical growth of children in the United States using data collected by the NCHS between 1963 and 1975.[6] This was done by examining a group of children chosen by a nationwide probability sample designed by the NCHS and the United States Bureau of Census. The examination and measurement processes were standardized. Careful application of statistical sampling weights to the sample of more than 20,000 children resulted in an effective representation of all children in the United States to the age of 18 years. These growth charts are well accepted and widely used.

Using the NCHS data, Broselow determined the 50th percentile weight for many lengths and heights. This was translated to a measuring tape with spaces labeled with weights in kilograms instead of units of length. The appropriate doses for many resuscitation drugs, calculated from the estimated weight and the American Heart Association (AHA) recommendations,[7] are printed in each space.

Our multicenter study was undertaken to evaluate the accuracy of weights estimated by this tape.

Materials and Methods

Children from one week to 12 years old were enrolled in our study at five institutions, from August to October 1986. Data were collected on pediatric patients seen in the emergency department and outpatient clinics of Harbor UCLA Medical Center in Los Angeles; the ED of University Hospital in Jacksonville, Florida; the pediatric cardiology clinics at Hartford Hospital in Connecticut; the pediatric intensive care unit and clinic, University of North Carolina at Chapel Hill;

and in the operating suite at Children's Hospital of Philadelphia. Age (to the nearest month), sex, ethnic background, and diagnosis were recorded for each child.

Patients were weighed to the nearest 0.1 kg on either a table or upright scale, depending on ability to stand. Length (or height) was measured to the nearest 0.1 cm. A prototype of the Broselow Tape was used to measure the child's length in the recumbent position, from crown to heel. The study tapes were marked with 33 spaces, numbered from 1 to 33. Each space corresponded to an estimated weight in whole kilograms. The space on the tape into which the child's length fell was noted. The evaluators were blinded to the relationship between the numbered spaces on the tape and the estimated weight corresponding to the space.

After all data were collected, the estimated weight (tape weight), in whole kilograms, for each child was derived from the relationship between weight and length developed by Broselow. The estimated tape weight versus the actual weight were plotted, straight lines were fitted through the data using linear regression analysis, and the slopes of the resulting lines were analyzed. Comparisons of observed slopes with expected slopes were made with a t test. Error and percent error of the tape weight from the actual weight were calculated.

A comparison was made between the Broselow Tape and the most commonly used method, estimation of weight based on age. An additional group of 53 children between 1 month and 11 years old who were seen in the pediatric ED at Harbor-UCLA Medical Center were weighed and measured as described above by a single observer. The child's weight then was estimated by three separate individuals selected from a group of pediatric residents, emergency medicine residents, family medicine residents, and pediatric emergency nurses. The "estimators" were told the child's age and observed the child unclothed, sitting, and/or supine. Absolute values for the error and percent error were calculated; corresponding errors were obtained for the tape. The percent errors of the estimates were compared with those of the tape in a two-way contingency table, and the significance was evaluated using Fisher's exact test.

Results

The children in this study (N = 1,002) ranged in age from 2 weeks to 10 years, 11 months old, with 57% boys. There were no significant differences in the accuracy of the tape for boys versus girls or among ethnic groups. Accuracy for patients with chronic cardiac and neurologic disorders did not significantly differ from that for healthy and acutely ill children. As a result, the entire data set was pooled for analysis.

The weight of the population ranged from 2.05 to 51.10 kg, and length ranged from 43.00 to 145.10 cm. The increments on the tape begin at 53 cm, with the first space, number 1, corresponding to 4 kg. The last space, number 33, corresponds to an estimated weight of 36 kg. A number of children initially enrolled in this study exceeded the range of the tape in its prototype form, so the data for the children less than 3.5 kg and those greater than 40 kg were discarded. Tape weight versus actual weight was plotted for the remaining set of subjects (n = 937). When linear regression analysis (y = a + bx) was performed, the result was a line with the equation: tape weight = 1.01 + 0.89 (actual weight), r = 0.97.

The data were grouped into weight ranges for analysis. For subjects in the 3.5 to 10 kg range (n = 395), the slope of the regression line is 0.98 with r = 0.89. For children from 10 to 25 kg (n = 449), the slope of the regression line is 0.96 with r = 0.93. For those weighing more than 25 kg (n = 93), the slope falls off to 0.50 (r = 0.46). When these slopes are compared with the "ideal" slope of 1.0 by a two-tailed t test, the results are P = .28, P = .13, and P<.00001, respectively. This indicates that the slopes for the subjects between 3.5 and 25 kg do not significantly vary from 1.0, but in the group weighing more than 25 kg, there is significant deviation from the desired slope of 1.0.

The accuracy of the tape was further evaluated by looking at the error for each subject between the actual weight and the tape weight. The error (actual weight - tape weight) ranged from −5.7 kg to +15.7 kg, with a mean of +0.47 (SD = 1.93). This indicates that, on the average, the tape tends to underestimate the weight by approximately 0.5 kg. This is a statistically significant bias (P<.0001), but is usually not clinically important. The mean error is -0.05 kg (SD = 0.95) in the 3.5 to 10 kg group, 0.39 kg (SD = 1.62) in the 10 to 25 kg group, and 3.03 kg (SD = 3.67) in the more than 25 kg group.

The percent error was calculated for each subject. Almost 60% (59.7%) of all the tape estimates are within 10% of the true weight, and 79.2% are within ±15%. The percent error will necessarily be slightly more in the very young children, because every "space" (full-kilogram increments) away from the actual weight is a larger percentage of the whole (eg, if the tape estimates a 3.5-kg child to be 4 kg, the percent error is 14%, but this is as close as the tape can possibly be).

The slopes of the regression lines of actual versus tape-estimated weight for children less than 25 kg are not significantly different from the ideal slope of 1.00, but the accuracy significantly decreases for children weighing more than 25 kg. The decrease in accuracy above 25 kg may be exaggerated by the regression analysis data because of the small data set and considerable scatter. When the percent error is calculated for this group, 49.5% are within 10% of the true weight (59.7% for the entire data set). Another 21.5% are within 15% (cumulative 71%, compared with 79.2% for the entire set). The tape underestimated the actual weight by more than 20% in approximately 16% of these larger children. All of these children were noted by the evaluators to be obese.

The 53 children enrolled in the additional evaluation of the tape ranged between 1 month and 11 years old with weights from 4 to 31 kg. The absolute value of the errors for the tape weights ranged from 0 to 2.9 kg, with a mean of 0.66 kg (SD = 0.64). The errors for the weight estimates by residents and nurses ranged from 0.02 to 8.9 kg, with a mean of 1.85 kg (SD = 1.87). The tape weights are more often within 15% of the actual weight than the weights estimated by residents and nursing staff (94% vs 63%; P<.0001 by Fisher's exact test).

Discussion

Dosages of drugs and fluids given during pediatric emergencies and resuscitation are calculated on per kilogram basis. Several methods have been developed to rapidly estimate body weight. Today's most popular methods use age-specific weights, either memorized or obtained from a reference chart.[2] This requires recall and/or immediate access to a chart. There are other factors that may contribute to the inaccuracy of age-specific weights. If the age is unknown, both age and weight must be estimated; the interval between memorized values is often wide; and normal weights for a given age may vary widely, especially for older children.

Recently, relationships between length and weight have been explored as a source of weight estimation. Length is a readily obtainable measurement, even in the setting of CPR. Length is strongly related to many biologic processes such as glomerular filtration rate and intestinal absorption, and is a stronger determinant of body surface area than is weight.[4] Methods to generate ideal body mass as a function of height in adults were found to be useful in the determination of the doses of drugs that primarily distribute to the fat-free mass.[8]

A complicated formula for estimating ideal body mass from length in children was developed by Traub and Kichen.[4] They defined the 50th percentile weight for height from the NCHS data as "ideal" because it represents a child with average amounts of lean and adipose tissue for a given height. Their equation loses accuracy in taller children (especially those more than 154 cm tall). It was hypothesized that this was secondary to the exclusion of body frame as a variable in older children and the increasing percentage of body fat. It is likely that the ideal weight will more accurately reflect the actual weight in younger children and infants because of their increased amount of total body water and lower percentages of body fat.[9] This same 50th percentile measurement was used by Broselow in the development of the tape tested in our study.

Garland and coworkers in Milwaukee developed a method for estimating body weight from height and body habitus.[3]

With this method, slim, average, and heavy children are those whose weights are taken from the 5th, 50th, and 95th percentile for their heights. After height is measured and habitus determined, the estimated weight is obtained from a chart. In their study of 258 children, regression analysis of the actual versus estimated weight yielded a line with a slope of 1.04 when the regression line was forced through the origin (ie, an equation of the form y = bx). They also found that 61% of the estimates were within 10% error. A stepwise multiple regression was performed, and they determined that length was the most important variable in estimating weight, followed by body habitus, and then age.

In our study, a regression line with a slope of 0.95 was obtained when the regression line was forced through the origin (n = 937), and 59.7% of the estimates were within ±10%, with 79.2% within ±15%. The tape is as accurate as the method developed by Garland and associates and is easier to use because there is only one variable. There is no need for the memorization of drug dosages or the performance of calculations because the dosages recommended by the AHA are already calculated and presented on the tape. The addition of an interval corresponding to 3 kg would further increase the utility of this tape.

The decrease in accuracy of the tape demonstrated in our study for children weighing more than 25 kg was most likely due to the variations in weight and body habitus of these older children. Our data do show the increased scatter in this group. This decrease in accuracy of more than 25 kg is of concern, and perhaps modification to include body habitus as a variable at the higher weights should be considered.

The tape also was shown to be significantly more accurate than those weight estimates made from age and observation by residents and pediatric nurses, indicating its superiority over the method most commonly used today.

Conclusion

The method of weight estimation used by the Broselow Tape is highly accurate, matching or surpassing other methods already common or proposed for use. The tape provides a rapid, accurate method of estimating weight and the necessary drug dosages for critically ill and injured children. The need for memorization and calculation, which are major sources of human error in pediatric weight estimation and drug dosage calculations, is eliminated. The Broselow Tape is easy to use and should prove useful to both prehospital and ED health care providers.

References

1. Trussell J, Bloom DE: A model distribution of height or weight at a given age. *Human Biology*. 1979;51:523-536

2. Task Force on Pediatric Emergency Medicine: Workbook for Advanced Pediatric Life Support (APLS). Chapel Hill, NC: American Academy of Pediatrics. 1984:74

3. Garland JS, Kishaba RG, Nelson DB, et al. A rapid and accurate method of estimating body weight. *Am J Emerg Med*. 1986;4:390-393

4. Traub SL, Kichen L: Estimating ideal body mass in children. *Am J Hosp Pharm*. 1983;40:107-110

5. Broselow J, personal communication, July, 1986

6. Hamill PVV, Drizd TA, Johnson CL, et al. Physical growth: National Center for Health Statistics Percentiles. *Am J Clin Nutr*. 1979;32:607-629

7. Standards and guidelines for cardiopulmonary resuscitation and emergency cardiac care. *JAMA*. 1986;255: 2905-2984

8. Durnin JV, Womersley J: Body fat assessed from total body density and its estimation from skinfold thickness. *Br J Nutr*. 1974;32: 77-97

9. Ellis D, Avner ED: Fluid and electrolyte disorders in pediatric patients, in Purschett PB (ed): *Disorders of Fluid and Electrolyte Balance*. New York, NY: Churchill Livingstone; 1985:217-229

APPENDIX J

AMERICAN ACADEMY OF PEDIATRICS
Committee on Pediatric Emergency Medicine

ACCESS TO EMERGENCY MEDICAL CARE

More than 60,000 children seek emergency care each day in the United States. However, inequities in our present health care system often preclude the prompt and appropriate access to emergency care necessary to treat these infants, children, and young adolescents—hereafter referred to as children. Several important obstacles exist. (1) As of 1990, there were over 12 million uninsured American children.[1] (2) Many children are declared uninsurable because of chronic illnesses, disabling conditions, or other preexisting conditions. (3) Although emergency departments are required to evaluate all patients who seek care, it is well known that lack of insurance can serve as an obstacle to prompt access, transport to, and treatment at appropriate level emergency and critical care facilities. (4) There is not yet universal availability and appropriate use of the 911 access number.[2] (5) The extent to which pediatrics is included in the educational and training content of paramedic and basic emergency medical technician programs has been shown to be less than adequate.[3,4] (6) Finally, children have specialized needs, requiring services not always available in every hospital. Therefore, the obstacles to prompt access are magnified at a critical time for the child seeking emergency care.

Several recent developments have increased the recognition and understanding of the unique emergency medical care needs of children. These include: (1) the development of pediatric emergency medicine as a subspecialty of pediatrics (American Board of Pediatrics) and emergency medicine (American Board of Emergency Medicine); (2) the development of the American Academy of Pediatrics

(AAP)/American College of Emergency Physicians Advanced Pediatric Life Support course and the AAP/American Heart Association Pediatric Advanced Life Support course; (3) the federal Emergency Medical Services for Children grants; (4) the development of guidelines for Emergency Medical Services for Children[5]; and Institute of Medicine Studies under way to evaluate emergency care for children in the US.

The American Academy of Pediatrics recommends that every child in need of emergency care deserves access to optimal emergency services, without regard to socioeconomic status.[6] Efforts must be directed on local, state, and federal levels: (1) to increase public, professional, and governmental awareness about the magnitude of the problem of access to emergency care for children; (2) to fund, support, and promote the further development and improvement of Emergency Medical Services for Children; (3) to encourage all emergency departments to establish transfer agreements with tertiary care referral centers to assure access to care for critically ill and injured children; and (4) to guarantee prompt and appropriate access to emergency care for all children regardless of socioeconomic status, ethnic origin, geographic location, or health status.

There must be a national commitment to ensure access to quality emergency health care for all children.

Committee on Pediatric Emergency Medicine, 1991-1992

Stephen Ludwig, MD, Chairperson
J. Alexander Haller, Jr, MD
Marc L. Holbrook, MD
Jane Knapp, MD
William J. Lewander, MD
James S. Seidel, MD, PhD
Calvin C.J. Sia, MD
Jonathan Singer, MD
Joseph A. Weinberg, MD

Liaison Representatives

Max L. Ramenofsky, MD
American College of Surgeons
Robert W. Schafermeyer, MD
American College of Emergency Physicians

AAP Section Liaisons

Daniel Notterman, MD
Section on Critical Care
James O'Neill, MD
Section on Surgery

References

1. Employee Benefit Research Institute. "Sources of Health Insurance and Characteristics of the Uninsured: Analysis of the March 1991 Current Population Survey." *EBRI Issue Brief.* 1992;123
2. Seidel JS, Henderson DP, eds. *Emergency Medical Services for Children: A Report to the Nation.* Washington, DC: National Center for Education In Maternal and Child Health; 1991.
3. Seidel JS. Emergency medical services and the pediatric patient: are the needs being met? II: training and equipping emergency medical service providers for pediatric emergencies. *Pediatrics.* 1986;78:808-812
4. Seidel JS, Hornbein M, Yoshiyama K, Kuznets D, Finklestein JZ, St. Geme JW. Emergency medical services and the pediatric patient: are the needs being met? *Pediatrics.* 1984;73:769-772
5. American Medical Association Commission on Emergency Medical Services. Pediatric Emergencies. *Pediatrics.* 1990;85:879-887
6. Strain JE. The American Academy of Pediatrics Response to the Growing Health Needs of Children. *Am J Dis Child.* 1991;145:536-539

APPENDIX K

SAMPLE

TRANSFER AGREEMENT BETWEEN REFERRAL HOSPITAL, INC. AND _____

To facilitate the transfer of patients between _____ Hospital (hereafter referred to as "_____") and Referral Hospital, Inc. the following procedures are set forth and agreed upon by the two institutions. The guiding principle of these procedures is to protect the best interest of the patient while transferring the patient from one institution to another.

1. The decision to transfer a patient shall be made jointly between the attending physician or his or her designate at _____ and the receiving physician or his or her designate at Referral Hospital, Inc. This decision will assure that adequate facilities are available at Referral Hospital, Inc. for a patient who is properly prepared for the transfer.

2. A copy of the complete medical record, including x-rays and laboratory reports, must be transferred with the patient. In addition, the following information should be available prior to the patient's transfer: (a) medical authorization; (b) patient's or guardian's consent; and (c) proper patient identification.

3. Patients who require a *burn unit* for their inpatient care shall not be transferred to Referral Hospital, Inc.

4. The physician sending the patient and the appropriate physician at Referral Hospital, Inc. shall consult regarding the necessity for medical or support personnel to accompany the patient and the appropriate mode of transportation. (Land ambulance or heli-

copter.) However, the final decision shall be that of the referring physician.

5. When a patient does not require a physician to accompany the patient, _____ shall provide appropriate support personnel during the transfer. In this case, the source and mode of transportation should consider returning personnel to _____.

6. When a physician from Referral Hospital, Inc. does not accompany the patient in transit, _____ shall assume medical responsibility for the patient until the patient arrives at the Emergency Services of Referral Hospital, Inc. Upon such arrival, Referral Hospital, Inc. will assume medical responsibility for the patient.

7. When a physician from Referral Hospital, Inc. accompanies the patient in transit, Referral Hospital, Inc. shall assume joint medical responsibility for the patient once the patient has been determined clinically stable for transportation and has departed from _____. Upon arrival at the Emergency Service of Referral Hospital, Inc. Referral Hospital, Inc. will assume medical responsibility for the patient.

8. Referral Hospital, Inc. is not responsible for any costs associated with the transportation of a patient by land or by air. Such costs shall be billed by the organization providing the transportation to the responsible party of the patient.

9. _____ will initiate a transfer by calling Referral Hospital's 1-800-333-3333 referral line. Referral Hospital, Inc. will contact the physician closest from that day's on-call list by the referring physician. The physician or her or his designate (another physician) will return the referring physician's call promptly. A nurse from the referring hospital will call a nursing report to the appropriate receiving nurse at Referral Hospital, Inc. based upon expected _____ area.

10. Referral Hospital, Inc. and its physicians agree to provide appropriate information to the referring physician and hospital about the progress and disposition of the patient after the transfer is completed and for the duration of the patient's stay.

11. Referral Hospital, Inc. agrees to accept patients under age 18 years without regard for the patient's financial or third-party funding status within known hospital resources and accommodations.

12. _____ agrees to make the decision regarding the transfer to Referral Hospital, Inc. versus admitting the patient or transferring to another institution without regard for the patient's financial or third-party funding.

13. In the event either party in its own unilateral judgment determines to perform under this agreement and corrective efforts made in good faith by both parties are unsuccessful, either party may terminate this agreement upon the giving of 30 days' prior written notice without penalty.

14. This agreement shall be in effect for a period of 1 year beginning on the date of signature below. It shall be automatically renewed on an annual basis unless either party expresses its intent in writing to terminate or renegotiate the agreement at least 60 days prior to the renewal date.

Director of Emergency Services, Referral Hospital, Inc.	
Administrator Referral Hospital, Inc.	Administrator
(Date)	(Date)

APPENDIX L

SUMMARY OF STATE AND TERRITORY LAWS AFFECTING CARE OF MINORS

State	Age of Majority*	Emancipation Provisions†	Statute of Limitations (in y)	Maximum Period in Which to Bring Suit (If Different From S of L)	Statute of Limitations for Minors	Exception to Maximum for Minors
Alabama	19	Yes	2 (or 6 mo after injury discovered or should have been)	4 y	Same as adult	If under 4, until 8th birthday
Alaska	18	Yes	2	•••	Majority + 2 y	•••
Arizona	18	Yes	3 (from injury or, if object or intentional concealment or misrepresentation, when object or injury discovered)	•••	Up to age 7 + 3 y or on death + 3 y	•••
Arkansas	18	Yes	2	•••	Majority + 2 y	•••
California	18	Yes	3 (from injury or 1 y after discovered or should have been, whichever less)	•••	Majority + 3 y	•••

State	Age of Majority*	Emancipation Provisions†	Statute of Limitations (in y)	Maximum Period in Which to Bring Suit (If Different From S of L)	Statute of Limitations for Minors	Exception to Maximum for Minors
Colorado	21	Common law rules govern	2 (from discovered or should have been)	3 y (after act)	Majority + 2 y	•••
Connecticut	18	No	2	3 y (if injury results in death)	Same as adult	•••
Delaware	18	Yes	2 (from injury or when discovered)	3 y (after injury)	Same as adult	If under 6, until 6th birthday
DC	18	No	3	•••	Majority + 3 y	•••
Florida	18	No	2 (from discovered or should have been)	•••	Same as adult	•••
Georgia	18	Yes	2	•••	Majority + 2 y	•••
Hawaii	18	Yes	2 (from discovered or should have been)	6 y (from act)	Majority + 2 y	•••

State	Age of Majority*	Emancipation Provisions†	Statute of Limitations (in y)	Maximum Period in Which to Bring Suit (If Different From S of L)	Statute of Limitations for Minors	Exception to Maximum for Minors
Idaho	18	Yes	2 (from act) NB: If object left in body, or in case of fraud, then from discovery + 1 y (whichever later)	•••	Majority + 2 y	6 y
Illinois	18	Yes	2 (from discovered or should have been)	4 y	Majority + 2 y	8 y
Indiana	18	No	2 (from act)	•••	Same as adult, eg, if under 6, until 8th birthday	•••
Iowa	18	No	2	•••	Majority + 1 y	•••
Kansas	18	Yes	2 (from discovered or should have been)	4 y (from act)	Majority + 1 y	8 y
Kentucky	18	Yes	1 (from discovered or should have been)	•••	Majority + 1 y	•••
Louisiana	18	Yes	1 (from occurrence or discovery)	3 y (from occurrence)	Same as adult	•••

State	Age of Majority*	Emancipation Provisions†	Statute of Limitations (in y)	Maximum Period in Which to Bring Suit (If Different From S of L)	Statute of Limitations for Minors	Exception to Maximum for Minors
Maine	18	Yes	2	•••	Majority + 2 y	•••
Maryland	18	Yes	5 (from act) 3 (from discovery) whichever shorter	Time period begins at age 11, 16 if reproductive organs injured	16 + 5 y (from act) 3 y (from discovery) whichever shorter	•••
Massachusetts	18	Yes	7	•••	Same as adult, eg, if under 9 until 9th birthday	7 y
Michigan	18	Yes	2 (from act) 6 mo (from discovered or should have been)	•••	Majority + 1 y	•••
Minnesota	18	No	2	•••	Majority + 1 y	7 y
Mississippi	21	No	2 (from discovered or should have been)	•••	16 + 2 y	•••

State	Age of Majority*	Emancipation Provisions†	Statute of Limitations (in y)	Maximum Period in Which to Bring Suit (If Different From S of L)	Statute of Limitations for Minors	Exception to Maximum for Minors
Missouri	18	No	2 (from act) NB: If object left in body, then from discovery + 2 y	10 y (from act)	If under 10, until 12th birthday	•••
Montana	18	Yes	3 (from discovered or should have been)	5 y (from injury)	If under 4, statute begins at 8 y	•••
Nebraska	19	Yes	2	•••	Same as adult	•••
Nevada	18	Yes	2 (from discovered or should have been)	•••	Same as adult, eg, for brain damage (until 10) or sterility (discovery + 2 y)	•••
New Hampshire	18	No	3	•••	Majority + 2 y	•••
New Jersey	18	No	2	•••	Majority + 2 y	•••
New Mexico	18	Yes	3 (from act)	•••	Same as adult, eg, if under 6, until 9th birthday	•••

State	Age of Majority*	Emancipation Provisions†	Statute of Limitations (in y)	Maximum Period in Which to Bring Suit (If Different From S of L)	Statute of Limitations for Minors	Exception to Maximum for Minors
New York	18	No	2½	•••	Majority + 2½ y	•••
North Carolina	18	Yes	3 (from act) 1 (from discovered or should have been, or from discovery of foreign object)	4 y 10 y (foreign object)	Same as adult	•••
North Dakota	18	Yes	2 (from discovered or should have been)	6 y	Majority + 1 y	12 y
Ohio	18	Yes	1	•••	Within 4 y of occurrence, eg, if under 10, until 14th birthday	•••
Oklahoma	18	No	2 (from discovered or should have been)	•••	Majority + 1 y	If under 12 within 7 y

State	Age of Majority*	Emancipation Provisions†	Statute of Limitations (in y)	Maximum Period in Which to Bring Suit (If Different From S of L)	Statute of Limitations for Minors	Exception to Maximum for Minors
Oregon	18	Yes	2 (from discovered or should have been) or in case of fraud, when discovered or should have been	5 y Except fraud	Same as adult	...
Pennsylvania	21	Yes	2	...	Same as adult	...
Puerto Rico	21	Yes	1	...	Same as adult	...
Rhode Island	18	Common law followed	3	...	Majority + 3 y	...
South Carolina	18	No	3 (from reasonable discovery)	6 y	Majority + 1 y	...
South Dakota	18	Yes	2	...	Majority + 1 y	...
Tennessee	18	No	1	...	Majority + 1 y	...
Texas	18	Yes	2	...	Majority + 2 y	...

State	Age of Majority*	Emancipation Provisions†	Statute of Limitations (in y)	Maximum Period in Which to Bring Suit (If Different From S of L)	Statute of Limitations for Minors	Exception to Maximum for Minors
Utah	18	Yes	2 (from discovered or should have been) 1 (from discovery of fraud or object)	4 years (from act) except fraud or object	Same as adult	•••
Vermont	18	No	3	•••	Majority + 3 y	•••
Virginia	18	No	2	•••	Majority + 2 y	•••
Virgin Islands	18	Yes	2	•••	21 + 2 y	•••
Washington	18	No	3 (from act) 1 (from discovered or should have been, whichever later)	8 years (from act)	Majority + 3 y	•••
West Virginia	21	Yes	2	•••	Majority + 2 y	No more than 20 years
Wisconsin	18	Yes	3 (from act) 1 (from discovered or should have been, whichever later)	•••	Same as adult, eg, if under 10 until 10th birthday (whichever later)	•••

State	Age of Majority*	Emanci-pation Provisions†	Statute of Limitations (in y)	Maximum Period in Which to Bring Suit (If Different From S of L)	Statute of Limitations for Minors	Exception to Maximum for Minors
Wyoming	19	Common law governs	2 (from act or discovery)	•••	Same as adult, eg, if under 8	•••

Adapted from *Martindale Hubbel Law Directory*, 1991. Information on this chart reflects state-by-state statutory provisions for negligence and medical malpractice actions. Provisions for each category may be different for other purposes and causes of action.

*For purposes of consent generally and period of disability (ie, minority) for medical malpractice actions.

†Characteristically *marriage, court decree by petition, armed services*. States whose statutes do not speak to the issue of emancipation *per se* may have provisions under which disabilities of minority may be removed: see state statute.

APPENDIX M

MEDICAL DIAGNOSTIC CHILD ABUSE PROGRAMS IN THE UNITED STATES AND CANADA

Compiled by The American Academy of Pediatrics Section on Child Abuse and Neglect, June 1991

Introduction

The following listing was developed by the Section on Child Abuse and Neglect of the American Academy of Pediatrics in response to requests for medical diagnostic programs in the United States that practitioners can use for referral. The Section on Child Abuse offers no recommendations nor endorsements of these programs. Responsibility lies with the referent to see that a particular program matches the patients' needs.

Those medical programs wishing to be included should send a one paragraph description of the program along with its name, address, phone number, and medical director to: Laura Aird, Sections Coordinator, Section on Child Abuse and Neglect, American Academy of Pediatrics, 141 Northwest Point Blvd, PO Box 927, Elk Grove Village, IL 60009-0927.

Lawrence R. Ricci, MD
Chairperson
Section on Child Abuse and Neglect
American Academy of Pediatrics
July 1, 1991

Alabama

Bessemer Child Advocacy Center
District Attorney Samuel Russell
Courthouse Annex
Bessemer, AL 35020-4907
205/481-4145
Director: Harold Johnston

Arizona

Maricopa Medical Center
Child Advocacy Program
PO Box 5099
Phoenix, AZ 85010
602/267-5404
Director: Mary Rimsza, MD

The Child Abuse Prevention Center of St Joseph's Hospital
350 W Thomas Rd
Phoenix, AZ 85013
602/285-3621
Director: Kay Rauth-Farley, MD
602/285-3716

Dept of Pediatrics Evaluation Clinic
University of Arizona College of Medicine
Tucson, AZ 85724
602/626-6303
Director: Anna Binhiewicz, MD

Arkansas

Program for Children at Risk
Arkansas Children's Hospital
800 Marshall St
Little Rock, AR 72202
501/320-1013
Director: Jerry G. Jones, MD

California

FHP Health Care
818 W Alondra Bvd
Compton, CA 90220
213/537-1337
Director: Lillie Williams, MD
213/496-4900

Childhood Sexual Abuse Evaluation Program
Valley Medical Center
445 S Cedar Ave
Fresno, CA 93702
209/453-5758
Director: Joyce Adams, MD

Children's Protection Center
Memorial Miller Children's Hospital
2801 Atlantic Ave
Long Beach, CA 90801-1426
213/595-2555
Director: Mark H. Goodman, MD, FAAP
213/595-2555

Los Angeles County - University of Southern California
Medical Center for the Vulnerable Child
1129 N State St - Pediatrics
Los Angeles, CA 90033
213/226-3961
Director: Astrid H. Heger, MD

SCAN Team - Merrithew Memorial Hospital
2500 Alhambra Ave
Martinez, CA 94553
415/370-5000 or 415/370-5490
Director: Jim Carpenter, MD, MPH
415/370-5000

Sexual Abuse Management Clinic (SAM)
Children's Hospital Oakland
747 52nd St
Oakland, CA 94609
415/428-3000 X 2254
Director: James J. Williams, MD
415/428-3257

Child Abuse Services Team
401 City Drive S
Orange, CA 92668
714/935-6390
Director: Cathy Campbell
714/935-6788

Child Abuse and Neglect Team
Riverside General Hospital
9851 Magnolia Ave
Riverside, CA 92503
714/358-7561
Director: Clare Sheridan, MD
714/824-4304

Child Protection Center
University of California, Davis Medical Center
2315 Stockton Blvd, Trailer 1531
Sacramento, CA 95817
916/734-8396
Director: Marilyn Peterson, MSW, MPA
Medical Director: Michael Reinhard, MD
916/734-3453

Children in Crisis Center
St Bernardine Medical Center
2101 N Waterman Ave
San Bernardino, CA 92404
714/881-4321
Director: Herbert A. Giese, MD, MPH, FAAP
714/881-4321

Children's Hospital & Health Center
Center for Child Protection
8001 Frost St
San Diego, CA 92131
619/576-5814
Director: David L. Chadwick, MD

Center for Child Protection
Santa Clara Valley Medical Center
Department of Pediatrics
751 S Bascom Ave
San Jose, CA 95128
408/299-6460
Director: David L. Kerns, MD
408/299-5562

San Luis Obispo County Suspected Abuse Response Team
2180 Johnson Ave
PO Box 8113
San Luis Obispo, CA 93403-8113
805/549-4878
Director: Jane A. Kulick, RN, PHN
805/549-4896

SART/SANE Program
Dominican Hospital
155 Soquel Dr
Rm 110
Santa Cruz, CA 95065
408/462-7744
Director: Sherry Arndt, RN, PHN

Harbor/UCLA Medical Center
1000 W Carson St
Bin 437
Torrance, CA 90509
213/533-3091
Directors: Carol Berkowitz, MD, James Seidel, MD, PhD

SCAN Team
Kaiser Walnut Creek
1425 S Main St
Walnut Creek, CA 94596
415/943-3491
Director: Walter Keller, MD

Canada
Hospital Child Abuse Committee
Sarnia General Hospital
220 Mitton St N
Sarnia, Ontario, Canada
519/383-8180
Director: Kunwar R. Singh, MD, FRCP, FAAP
519/336-6311

Child Protection Service Unit
BC Children's Hospital
4480 Oak St
Vancouver, BC, Canada, V6H3V4
604/875-2345
Director: J. Hlady, MD
604/875-2130

Colorado
C. Henry Kempe Natl Center for the
Prevention & Treatment of Child Abuse & Neglect
1205 Oneida St
Denver, CO 80220
303/321-3963
Director: Richard D. Krugman, MD

Child Advocacy and Protection Team
The Children's Hospital
1056 E 19th Ave
D-138
Denver, CO 80218
303/861-6919
Director: Carole Jenny, MD

Connecticut

Milford Hospital Emergency Department
2047 Bridgeport Ave
Milford, CT 06460
203/876-4100
Director: Jay Walshon, MD (Director, Emergency Medicine)

Hospital of Saint Raphael
Emergency Department
1450 Chapel St
New Haven, CT 06511
203/789-3464
Director: Paul Krochmal, MD

DART Committee
Yale-New Haven Hospital
Department of Pediatrics
c/o John M. Leventhal, MD
New Haven, CT
203/785-2468
Director: John M. Leventhal, MD

Florida

Child Protection Team
1901 Manatee Ave, W
Bradenton, Fl 34205
813/746-1904
Director: Diane Saunders

Child Protection Team (Satellite IB)
728 N Ferdon Blvd, Suite 5
Crestview, FL 32536
904/682-4688
Director: Edward H. Seeliger, MD

Child Protection Team
240 North Fredrick Ave
Daytona Beach, FL
904/238-3830
Director: Michael Bell, MD
904/734-1824

HRS-CMS District III, Child Protection Team
University of Florida
5700 SW 34th St
Suite 1310
Gainesville, FL 32608
904/392-7286
Director: F. Thomas Weber, MD
904/392-5960

Child Protection Team of the Children's Crisis Center, Inc
University Medical Center
655 W Eighth St
Jacksonville, FL 32209
904/366-2444
Director: J. M. Whitworth, MD
904/366-2456
CPT Medical Director: Bruce McIntosh, MD
904/387-7373

Center for Children in Crisis
1720 E Tiffany Dr
Mangonia Park, FL 33407-3223
407/863-1611
Director: Lawrence R. Leviton, MD
407/832-1139

Community Health of South Dade-Child Protection Team
10300 SW 216 St
Miami, FL 33190
305/252-4822
Directors: Barbara Lew, MD, Phyllis Harriet

Child Protection Team of Collier County
2500 Airport Rd
Suite 308
Naples, FL
813/263-2858
Director: Richard E. Marting, MD

Pasco Family Protection Team
7619 Little Rd
Suite 325 Counsel Square
New Port Richey, FL 34654
813/848-4878
Director: Andrew Gellady

Child Protection Team-District 7A
85 W Miller STE 304
Orlando, FL 32806
407/841-5111 X 5940
Director: Matthew Seibel, MD

Child Protection Team
2012 Lisenby Ave
Suite A
Panama City, FL 32405
904/763-8449
Director: Malcolm M. Traxler, MD
904/763-5413

Brevard County Child Protection Team
1260 S US 1, Suite 203
Rockledge, FL 32903
407/632-7107
Director: Donald H. Arnold, Richard K. O'Heir
407/636-3066

Child Protection Team
1750 17th St
Sarasota, FL 34234
813/365-1277
Director: Hal Hedley

Suncoast Child Protection Team, Inc
3601 34th St N
St Petersburg, FL 33713
813/527-5955
Director: Patricia Wallace

Child Protection Team
1126-B Lee Ave
Tallahassee, FL 32303
904/487-2838
Director: Sam Moorer, MD
904/877-6119

Georgia

Dooly Medical Center
Union St
Vienna, GA 31092
912/268-4141
Director: Larry Anderson

Hawaii

CPS Team
Kapiolani Medical Center
Rm 710
1319 Punahou St
Honolulu, HI 96826
808/944-9940
Director: Steven J. Choy, PhD
808/944-9940

Idaho

CARES PROGRAM
St Lukes RMC
190 E Bammock
Boise, ID 83712
208/386-3063
Director: Tom Cornwall, MD

Illinois

Child Protection Team - Carle Clinic
Carle Clinic
602 W University Ave
Urbana, IL 61801
217/337-3100
Director: Kathleen Buetow, MD
217/337-3100

Protective Service Team
Children's Memorial Hospital
2300 Children's Plaza, Box 16
Chicago, IL 60614
312/880-3831
Director: Katherine Christoffel, MD, Edward Zieserl, MD

Columbus Cabrini Medical Center
2520 N Lakeview
Chicago, IL 60614
312/883-5908
Director: Emalee Flaherty, MD

Combined La Rabida - University of Chicago
Child Abuse and Neglect Program
East 65th St at Michigan
Chicago, IL 60649
312/363-6700
Director: Paula K. Jaudes, MD
312/363-6700 X 330

Pediatric Ecology Program
Mount Sinai Hospital Medical Center
Dept of Pediatrics
California Ave at 15th St
Chicago, IL 60608
312/650-6721
Director: Howard B. Levy, MD
312/650-6430

Indiana

Child Sexual Abuse Program
Indiana University
Department of Pediatrics
702 Barnhill Dr
Indianapolis, IN 46202
317/630-6920
Director: Roberta Ann Hibbard, MD
317/274-8271

Pediatric Advocates
285 W 12th
Peru, IN 46970
317/472-4356
Director: Neil J. Stalker, MD
317/472-4356

Iowa

Child Protection Center
St Lukes Hospital
1026 A Ave NE
Cedar Rapids, IA
319/369-8700
Director: Kathleen Opdebeeck, MD
319/369-8700

Family Ecology Center
1111 9th St
Des Moines, IA 50314
515/280-1808
Director: Rizwan Z. Shah, MD, FAAP

University of Iowa Child Abuse Program
University of Iowa
209 Hospital School
Iowa City, IA 52242
319/353-6136
Director: Randall Alexander, MD, PhD

Kansas
University of Kansas Medical Center
Dept of Pediatrics
39th & Rainbow
Kansas City, KS 66103
913/588-5908
Director: Lynn K. Sheets, MD

Kentucky
Department of Pediatrics/Kosair Children's Hospital
231 E Chestnut St
Louisville, KY 40202
502/629-7212
Director: Mary A. Smith, MD
502/629-7225

Louisiana
Child Sexual Abuse Program
Children's Hospital
200 Henry Clay
New Orleans, LA
504/896-9237
Director: Rebecca Rusell, MD

Maine
The Diagnostic Program for Child Abuse
Mid-Maine Medical Center
Waterville, ME 04901
207/872-4286
Director: Lawrence R. Ricci, MD

Maryland

CARE Clinic
700 W Lombard St
Baltimore, MD 21201
301/328-5176
Director: Howard Dubowitz, MD
301/328-5289

SAFE Clinic (Sexual Abuse Follow-Up & Evaluation)
Mercy Medical Center
301 St Paul Pl
Baltimore, MD 21202
301/332-9351
Director: Charles I. Shubin, MD

Massachusetts

Boston City Hospital Child Protection Program
818 Harrison Ave
Boston, MA 02118
617/534-4503
Director: Jan Paradise, MD

Child Protection Program
Children's Hospital
Boston, MA 02115
617/735-7979
Director: Eli H. Newberger, MD

Brockton Children and Youth Project
Family Violence Consultation Group
680 Centre St
Brockton, MA 02402
508/583-2900
Director: John J. McNamara, MD

Family Advocacy Project
Bay State Medical Center, 140 High St
Springfield, MA 01199
413/784-5083
Director: Edward N. Bailey, MD

Child Advocacy Team and Family Center Project
University of Massachusetts Medical Center
55 Lake Ave N
Worcester, MA 01655
508/856-6629
Director: Deborah Madansky, MD
508/856-3281

Michigan

Grace Hospital Child Protection Program
6071 W Outer Dr, Suite L541
Detroit, MI 48235
Clinical Coordinator: Mary Stanley Lawson
313/966-3133
Director: Dr Ceres Morales
313/966-3133

Project Harmony
Kent County Council for the Prevention of Child Abuse
  and Neglect
161 Ottawa NW
Grand Rapids, MI 49503
616/454-4673
Coordinator: Carol Bennett
616/454-4614

Great Lakes Pediatrics Associates
4031 W Main St #100
Kalamazoo, MI 49007
616/342-9313
Director: David K. Hickok, MD, FAAP
616/342-9313

Child Protecting Team
900 Woodward
Pontiac, MI 48053
313/858-3000
Director: A. Church, MD
313/858-300

Minnesota

Mayo Clinic Child Abuse Team
200 First St SW
Rochester, MN 55905
507/284-2511
Director: Julia A. Rosekrans, MD
507/255-5388

Midwest Children's Resource Center
360 Sherman St
Suite 200
St Paul, MN 35102
612/220-6750
Director: Carolyn Levitt, MD
612/220-5040

Missouri

University of MO Child Abuse Evaluation Program
Dept of Child Health
Univ of MO Hospital
Columbia, MO 65212
314/882-4730
Director: Teresa Esquivel, MD
314/882-4730

New Jersey

Jersey Shore Medical Center
Child Abuse Diagnostic Center
C/O Social Work Department
1945 Route 33
Neptune, NJ 07754
908/776-4245
Director: Joseph Bogdan, MD
908/776-4245

Child Protective Committee -UMDNJ. RWJ Medical School
St Peter's Medical Center
Dept of Pediatrics
254 Eastern Ave
New Brunswick, NJ 08903
201/745-8600 ext 8783
Director: Kim K. Cheng, MD
Director for Sexual Abuse Program: Linda Shaw, MD
201/418-3146

Center for Children's Support-A Resource for the Evaluation
   and Treatment of Child Sexual Abuse
University of Medicine and Dentistry of NJ
School of Osteopathic Medicine
301 S Central Plaza, Suite 2100
Stratford, NJ 08084
609/346-7036
Director: Martin A. Finkel, DO, Medical Director
Esther Deblinger, PhD, Clinical Director

Sexual Abuse Management Clinic
Suite G, Robert Wood Johnson V. Hospital, UMDNJ
One RWJ Pl
New Brunswick, NJ 08903-0019
201/418-3133
Director: Linda Shaw, MD, MSW
201/418-3146

New York

Norman S. Ellenstein Child Abuse Center
Children's Hospital of Buffalo
219 Bryant St
Buffalo, NY 14222
716/878-7109
Director: Allan E. Korrberg, MD
716/878-7109

Crisis Nursery-New York Foundling Hospital
590 Avenue of the Americas
New York, NY 10011
212/472-8555
Director: Vincent J. Fontana, MD
212/886-4050

Family Advocacy Program
Jacobi Hospital
Pelham Parkway
Bronx, NY 10461
212/918-4568
Co Directors: Kathleen Porder, MD, and Jamie Roesenfeld, MD
212/918-4568

Mt Sinai Medical Center
Division of Ambulatory Pediatrics
Box 1160
New York, NY 10029
212/241-7156
Director: Katherine Teets Grimm, MD

The New York Hospital-Cornell Medical Center
Program for the Prevention of Child Abuse
525 E 68th St
New York, NY 10021
212/746-3305
Director: Daniel B. Kessler, MD

Project CEASE (Comprehensive Evaluation of
    Abusive Sexual Events)
Dept of Pediatrics, ECMC
462 Grider St
Buffalo, NY 14215
716/898-4900
Director: Stephen Lazoritz, MD

Child Protection Team
Schneider Children's Hospital
New Hyde Park, NY 11042
718/470-3281
Director: Bruce N. Bogard, MD

Child Abuse Referral and Evaluation (CARE)
Dept Pediatrics
Suny Health Science Center
750 E Adams St
Syracuse, NY 13210
315/464-5420
Director: Celeste Madden, MD and Ann Botash, MD
315/464-4363 or 315/464-5800

North Carolina

Asheville Pediatric Association
77 McDowell St
Asheville, NC 28801
704/254-5326
Director: Andrea Gravatt, MD

Family Advocacy Program, US Navy
Naval Hospital, Dept of Pediatrics
Cherry Point, NC 28533
919/466-5751
Dept Head: LCDR. Anthony N. Mishik, MC, USNR
919/466-0245

Child Sexual Abuse Team
Wake AHEC
PO Box 14465
Raleigh, NC 27620-4465
919/250-8493
Director: V. Denise Everett, MD
919/250-8493

WNC Regional Child Abuse Center
PO Box 5861
Asheville, NC 28813
704/254-2000
Director: Beth Peterinelli

Ohio

Children at Risk Evaluation (CARE) Center
Children's Hospital Medical Center of Akron
281 Locust St
Akron, OH 44308
216/379-8453
Director: R. Daryl Steiner, DO

Social and Medical Clinic and Child Abuse Team
Children's Hospital Medical Center
3350 Elland Ave
Cincinnati, OH 45229-2899
513/559-4711
Director: Robert Shapiro, MD
513/559-4506

Child Protection Program
Rainbow Babies and Children's Hospital
University Hospitals of Cleveland
2074 Abington Rd
Cleveland, OH 44106
216/844-3761
Director: Robert M. Reece, MD

Child Abuse Program
Children's Hospital
700 Children's Dr
Columbus, OH 43205
614/461-2504
Director: Charles Felzen Johnson, MD

Child Abuse Review and Evaluation Team and Clinic
The Children's Medical Center
One Children's Plaza
Dayton, OH 45404-1815
513/226-8403
Director: Libby Caudill, MSW, LISW

Child and Family Assessment Unit
Medical College of Ohio
Toledo, OH 43699
419/381-4487
Director: W. David Gemmill, MD, MS

Oklahoma

University of Oklahoma College of Medicine-Tulsa
2815 S Sheridan
Tulsa, OK 74129
918/838-4843
Director: Robert W. Block, MD
918/838-4725

Oregon

Sacred Heart Hospital Sexual Abuse Evaluation Program
12th & Hillgard St
Eugene, OR 97401
503/687-0572
Director: Scott Halpert, MD

Lincoln City Medical Center, PC
2870 W Devils Lake Rd
Lincoln City, OR 97367
503/994-9191
Director: Robert D. Sewell, MD, FAAP
503/994-9191

Child Abuse Response and Evaluation Services
   (CARES) Program
Emanuel Hospital
2801 N Gantenbein St
Portland, OR 97227
503/280-4943
Director: Jan Bays, MD, FAAP

Pennsylvania

Pediatric Practices of Northeastern Pennsylvania
1837 Fair Ave
Honesdale, PA 18431
717/253-5838
Contact Physician: Paul Diamond, MD

CVMH Child Protection Team
1086 Franklin St
Johnstown, PA 15905
814/533-9000
Director: Lawrence Rosenberg, MD
814/536-8956

Children's Advocacy Center
1107 Wilmington Rd
New Castle, PA
412/658-4688
Director: David Evrard

Children's Hospital SCAN Team
Children's Hospital of Philadelphia
34th St and Civic Center Blvd
Philadelphia, PA 19104
215/590-2067
Director: Stephen Ludwig, MD
215/590-2162

Sunbury Community Hospital Center for Child Protection
Sunbury Community Hospital
Sunbury, PA 17801
717/286-3333
Director: P.J. Bruno, MD, FAAP
717/286-7754

South Carolina
Family Services Clinic
5 Richland Medical Park
Acc I, Area C
Columbia, SC 29203
803/765-7211
Director: Susan V. Breeland, MD
803/765-7211

Tennessee
Child Abuse Clinic
1924 Alcoa Highway
Knoxville, TN 37920
615/544-9327
Director: Melinda A. Lucus
615/544-9327

Memphis Sexual Assault Resource Center
2600 Poplar Ave
Suite 300
Memphis, TN 38112
904/528-2161
Manager: Mary Durham

"Our Kids" Vanderbilt Child Abuse Evaluation Program
Metro Nashville General Hospital
72 Hermilage Ave
Nashville, TN 37210
615/259-5111
Director: Robert Brayden, MD

Texas

Child Assessment Program
601 E 15th St
Austin, TX 78701
512/480-1828
Director: Beth Nauert, MD
512/443-4800

REACH CLINIC
Children Medical Center
1935 Motor St
Dallas, TX 75235
214/920-2296
Director: Paul R. Prescott, MD
214/920-2296

Child Advocacy, Research and Education (CARE) Center
Department of Pediatrics
Texas Tech University Health Sciences Center
3601 4th St
Lubbock, Texas 79430
806/743-2121
Director: Rafael R. Garcia, MD
806/743-2121

CASIS (Child and Adolescent Sexual Abuse Intervention Services)
Bexar County Hospital District
4502 Medical Dr
San Antonio, TX 78229
512/270-3652
Director: Nancy Kellogg, MD

Virginia

Child Advocacy Committee
Children's Hospital of The King's Daughters
800 W Olney Rd
Norfolk, VA 23508
804/628-7179
Director: John M. de Triquet, MD

Washington

Children's Protection Team
Children's Hospital & Medical Center
4800 Sand Point Way NE
PO Box C5371
Seattle, WA 98105
206/526-2000
Director: Jill Cole, MSW
206/526-2167

Harborview Sexual Assault Center
Harborview Medical Center ZA-07
325 9th Ave
Seattle, WA 98104
206/223-3047
Director: Mary Gibbons, MD

Sexual Assault Clinic and Child Abuse Program
Mary Bridge Children's Hospital & Health Center
311 S L St
Tacoma, WA 98405
206/594-1478
Medical Director: Robert Scherz, MD

Regional Center for Child Abuse and Neglect
Deaconess Medical Center
PO Box 248, Spokane, WA 99210-0248
509/623-7501
Director: Alan Hendrickson, MD
Manager: Mary Ann Murphy

West Virginia

West Virginia University - Charleston Division and
   Women and Children's Hospital Sexual Abuse Team
800 Pennsylvania Ave
Charleston, WV 25302
304/347-9338 (social services)
Director: Kathleen V. Previll, MD
304/342-8272

Wisconsin

Child Abuse/Neglect Evaluation
Marshfield Clinic
1000 N Oak St
Marshfield, WI 54449
715/387-5251
Director: Gerald E. Porter, MD
715/387-5251

APPENDIX N

AMERICAN ASSOCIATION OF POISON CONTROL CENTERS*

Certified Regional Poison Centers, April 1992

(The numbers listed in this appendix are current as of July 1992. The reader is advised to contact the local poison control center to update numbers frequently.)

Alabama
Regional Poison Control Center
The Children's Hospital of Alabama
1600 7th Ave South
Birmingham, AL 35233-1711
Emergency Phone: 205/939-9201
800/292-6678 (AL only) or 205/933-4050

Arizona
Arizona Poison and Drug Information Center
Arizona Health Sciences Center; Rm. #3204-K
1501 N Campbell Ave
Tucson, AZ 85724
Emergency Phone: 800/362-0101 (AZ only)
602/626-6016

Samaritan Regional Poison Center
Good Samaritan Regional Medical Center
1130 E McDowell, Suite A-5
Phoenix, AZ 85006
Emergency Phone: 602/253-3334

California
Fresno Regional Poison Control Center
of Fresno Community Hospital and Medical Center
2823 Fresno St
Fresno, CA 93721
Emergency Phone: 800/346-5922 or 209/445-1222

---

*Adapted with permission of the American Association of Poison Control Centers.

San Diego Regional Poison Center
UCSD Medical Center; 8925
225 Dickinson St
San Diego, CA 92103-8925
Emergency Phone: 619/543-6000
800/876-4766 (in 619 area code only)

San Francisco Bay Area Regional Poison
  Control Center
San Francisco General Hospital
1001 Potrero Ave, Building 80, Room 230
San Francisco, CA 94122
Emergency Phone: 415/476-6600

Santa Clara Valley Medical Center
  Regional Poison Center
751 South Bascom Ave
San Jose, CA 95128
Emergency Phone: 408/299-5112
800/662-9886 (CA only)

University of California, Davis, Medical
  Center Regional Poison Control Center
2315 Stockton Blvd
Sacramento, CA 95817
Emergency Phone: 916/734-3692
800/342-9293 (Northern CA only)

UCI Regional Poison Center
UCI Medical Center
101 The City Drive; Rt 78
Orange, CA 92668-3298
Emergency Phone: 714/634-5988
800/544-4404 (Southern CA Only)

Colorado
Rocky Mountain Poison and Drug Center
645 Bannock St
Denver, CO 80204
Emergency Phone: 303/629-1123

District of Columbia
National Capital Poison Center
Georgetown University Hospital
3800 Reservoir Rd, NW
Washington, DC 20007
Emergency Numbers: 202/625-3333
202/784-4660 (TTY)

Florida

The Florida Poison Information Center at
  Tampa General Hospital
PO Box 1289
Tampa, FL 33601
Emergency Phone: 813/253-4444 (Tampa)
800/282-3171 (Florida)

Georgia

Georgia Poison Center
Grady Memorial Hospital
80 Butler St SE
PO Box 26066
Atlanta, GA 30335-3801
Emergency Phone: 800/282-5846 (GA only)
404/589-4400

Indiana

Indiana Poison Center
Methodist Hospital of Indiana
1701 N Senate Blvd
PO Box 1367
Indianapolis, IN 46206-1367
Emergency Phone: 800/382-9097 (IN only)
317/929-2323

Kentucky

Kentucky Regional Poison Center of Kosair Children's Hospital
315 E Broadway
PO Box 35070
Louisville, KY 40232
Emergency Phone: 800/722-5725 (KY only)
502/629-7275

Maryland

Maryland Poison Center
20 N Pine St
Baltimore, MD 21201
Emergency Phone: 410/528-7701
800/492-2414 (MD only)

National Capital Poison Center (DC suburbs only)
Georgetown University Hospital
3800 Reservoir Rd, NW
Washington, DC 20007
Emergency Numbers: 202/625-3333
202/784-4660 (TTY)

Massachusetts
Massachusetts Poison Control System
300 Longwood Ave
Boston, MA 02115
Emergency Phone: 617/232-2120, 800/682-9211

Michigan
Blodgett Regional Poison Center
1840 Wealthy SE
Grand Rapids, MI 49506-2968
Emergency Phone: 800/632-2727 (MI only)
TTY 800/356-3232

Poison Control Center
Children's Hospital of Michigan
3901 Beaubien Blvd
Detroit, MI 48201
Emergency Phone: 313/745-5711

Minnesota
Hennepin Regional Poison Center
Hennepin County Medical Center
701 Park Ave
Minneapolis, MN 55415
Emergency Phone: 612/347-3141
Petline: 612/337-7387, TDD 612/337-7474

Minnesota Regional Poison Center
St Paul-Ramsey Medical Center
640 Jackson St
St Paul, MN 55101
Emergency Phone: 612/221-2113

Missouri
Cardinal Glennon Children's Hospital
  Regional Poison Center
1465 S Grand Blvd
St Louis, MO 63104
Emergency Phone: 314/772-5200, 800/366-8888

Montana
Rocky Mountain Poison and Drug Center
645 Bannock St
Denver, CO 80204
Emergency Phone: 303/629-1123

Nebraska

The Poison Center
8301 Dodge St
Omaha, NE 68114
Emergency Phone: 402/390-5555 (Omaha)
800/955-9119 (NE)

New Jersey

New Jersey Poison Information and Education System
201 Lyons Ave
Newark, NJ 07112
Emergency Phone: 800/962-1253

New Mexico

New Mexico Poison and Drug Information Center
University of New Mexico
Albuquerque, NM 87131-1076
Emergency Phone: 505/843-2551
800/432-6866 (NM only)

New York

Long Island Regional Poison Control Center
Nassau County Medical Center
2201 Hempstead Turnpike
East Meadow, NY 11554
Emergency Phone: 516/542-2323, 2324, 2325, 3813

New York City Poison Control Center
NYC Department of Health
455 First Ave, Room 123
New York, NY 10016
Emergency Phone: 212/340-4494, 212/P-O-I-S-O-N-S
TDD 212/689-9014

Ohio

Central Ohio Poison Center
700 Children's Dr
Columbus, OH 43205-2696
Emergency Phone: 614/228-1323, 800/682-7625
614/228-2272 (TTY), 614/461-2012

Cincinnati Drug & Poison Information Center
  and Regional Poison Control System
231 Bethesda Ave, ML 144
Cincinnati, OH 45267-0144
Emergency Phone: 513/558-5111
800/872-5111 (OH only)

Oregon

Oregon Poison Center
Oregon Health Sciences University
3181 SW Sam Jackson Park Rd
Portland, OR 97201
Emergency Phone: 503/494-8968
800/452-7165 (OR only)

Pennsylvania

Central Pennsylvania Poison Center
University Hospital
Milton S Hershey Medical Center
Hershey, PA 17033
Emergency Phone: 800/521-6110

The Poison Control Center
(serving the greater Philadelphia metropolitan area)
One Children's Center
Philadelphia, PA 19104-4303
Emergency Phone: 215/386-2100

Pittsburgh Poison Center
3705 Fifth Ave at DeSoto St
Pittsburgh, PA 15213
Emergency Phone: 412/681-6669

Rhode Island

Rhode Island Poison Center
593 Eddy St
Providence, RI 02903
Emergency Phone: 401/277-5727

Texas

North Texas Poison Center
5201 Harry Hines Blvd
PO Box 35926
Dallas, TX 75235
Emergency Phone: 214/590-5000
(TX only) 800/441-0040

Utah

Intermountain Regional Poison Control Center
50 North Medical Dr
Salt Lake City, UT 84132
Emergency Phone: 801/581-2151
800/456-7707 (UT only)

Virginia
Blue Ridge Poison Center
Box 67
Blue Ridge Hospital
Charlottesville, VA 22901
Emergency Phone: 804/925-5543, 800/451-1428

National Capital Poison Center (Northern VA only)
Georgetown University Hospital
3800 Reservoir Rd, NW
Washington, DC 20007
Emergency Numbers: 202/625-3333
202/784-4660 (TTY)

West Virginia
West Virginia Poison Center
3110 MacCorkle Ave SE
Charleston, WV 25304
Emergency Phone: 800/642-3625 (WV only)
304/348-4211

Wyoming
The Poison Center
8301 Dodge St
Omaha, NE 68114
Emergency Phone: 402/390-5555 (Omaha)
800/955-9119 (NE)

APPENDIX O

SIDS CENTERS LISTED BY STATE*

Alabama

† North Central Alabama Chapter
Lot 62, Cedar Grove Park
Maylene, AL 35114

Allison Ellison
President
(W) 205/663-0917
(H) 205/956-1963
Debra King
Referral Coordinator
(W) 205/592-1081

† South Central Alabama Chapter
3372 Buckboard Rd
Montgomery, AL 36116

David Knapp, MD
President
(W) 205/281-3130
(H) 205/244-0385

Bureau of Family Health
Services/Child Health Branch
434 Monroe St, Rm 381
Montgomery, AL 36130-1701

Doris Barnetto, MSW
Acting Director
(W) 205/261-5052

Alaska

Alaska SIDS Info & Counseling
Program
1231 Gambell St, Suite 302
Anchorage, AK 99501-4627

Linda Vlastuin, RN, MPH
Nursing Consultant
(W) 907/272-1534

Alaska Dept of Health & Social
Services
1231 Gambell St
Anchorage, AK 99501

Karen Pearson, RD, MD
Chief, Maternal & Child Health
(W) 907/274-7626

Arizona

† Arizona Chapter c/o Phoenix
Children's Hospital
909 E Brill
Phoenix, AZ 85006

Shirley Wagner
President
(W) 602/820-7408

---

* Adapted from the Sudden Infant Death Syndrome Alliance.
Resource Directory of SIDS Centers by State.
† Indicates State Chapters of the National Sudden Infant Death
Syndrome Alliance.

Office of Maternal & Child Health
1740 W Adams St, Rm 200
Phoenix, AZ 85007

Jane Pearson
Chief, Maternal & Child
    Health
(W) 602/542-1875

Arkansas

SIDS Information & Counseling
    Program
Arkansas Dept of Health
4815 W Markham
Little Rock, AR 72205-3867

Carolyn Beverly, MD, MPH
Medical Director
Debbie Frazier, RN
Project Coordinator
(W) 501/661-2199
(W) 501/661-2321

California

California SIDS Program
(CAPHND) PO Box 11447
Berkeley, CA 94701

Sally Jacober, MSW, MPH
Program Director
(W) 510/849-4111
(SIDS #) 800/369-7437 (in CA)

Guild for Infant Survival,
    Los Angeles County
2007 Brookport St
Covina, CA 91724

Dawn Lamb
President
(W) 818/961-2229

† Southern California Chapter
11384 Lorena Ln
El Cajon, CA 92020

Sally Saltzstein
President
(W) 619/440-4108

Guild for Infant Survival,
    Orange County
PO Box 17432
Irvine, CA 92713-7432

Lynne Trujillo
President
(W) 714/474-7437
(FAX) 714/968-7623

† Greater Los Angeles Chapter
3752 Motor Ave
Los Angeles CA 90406

Vicki Knight
President
(H) 310/398-7311
(W) 310/836-6664
(SIDS #) 310/663-6448
(SIDS #) 800/743-7452
    (LA only)
(FAX) 310/558-3713

International Guild for Infant
    Survival, Santa Clara County
424 Woodcock Ct
Milipitas, CA 95035

Howard & Sura Weiner
President
(W) 408/262-7607

† Central Coast of California Chapter
670 Romero Canyon Rd
Montecito, CA 93108

Sharon Palmer
President
(W) 805/565-3781

† Northern California Chapter
Children's Hospital & Medical
Center
747 52nd St
Oakland, CA 94609

Mary Elizabeth Lewis
President
(SIDS #) 510/428-3297
(H) 415/530-9542
(FAX) 510/450-0818

† Redwood Empire Contact
PO Box 1292
Rohnert Park, CA 94928

Marilyn Shappell
Area Contact
(H) 707/585-8582

Maternal & Child Health, State
Dept of Health
714 P St, Rm 750
Sacramento CA 95814

Rugmini Shah, MD
Director
(W) 916/323-8181

† Valley Sierra Chapter
4732 Crestwood Way
Sacramento, CA 95822

Paul Reiner
President
(W) 916/452-3981
(H) 209/369-7643

San Diego County Guild -
San Diegans Against SIDS
6244 Adobe Dr
San Diego, CA 92115

Peter Davis
President
(SIDS #) 619/222-9662

Riverside & San Bernardino Co
Guild for Infant Survival
14544 Pony Trail
Victorville, CA 92392

Kim Logsdon
Vice-President
(W) 619/951-0708

Colorado

CO Dept of Health - Medical
Affairs & Special Programs
4210 East 11th Ave
Denver, CO 80220

Robert McCurdy, MD
Director
(W) 303/331-8373

† Colorado SIDS Program, Inc
6825 E Tennessee Ave
Bldg 1, Suite 300
Denver, CO 80224-1631

Sheila Marquez, RN
Executive Director
(W) 303/320-7771
(SIDS #) 800/332-1018
(in CO only)
(FAX) 303/322-8775

Connecticut

† Hartford County Chapter
PO Box 14148
Hartford CT 06134

Donna Wnuck
President
Ann Carabillo
Referral Coordinator
(H) 203/684-4330
(H) 203/561-3271
(SIDS #) 203/684-6278
(FAX) 203/887-7309

Connecticut SIDS Info & Counseling
Program Connecticut -
State Dept of Health
150 Washington St
Hartford CT 06106

Jann Dalton, MSW
Project Director
(W) 203/566-3767

Maternal & Child Health -
State Dept of Health
150 Washington St
Hartford, CT 06106

John Sayers
Assistant Chief
(W) 203/566-2887

† Eastern Connecticut Chapter
9 Gonch Farm Rd (PO Box 338)
Ledyard, CT 06339

Charles Mihalko
President
(W) 203/447-1791 X 4541
(SIDS #) 203/889-8331
(FAX) 203/887-7309

† Fairfield/New Haven Chapter
275 Long Ridge Rd
Stamford CT 06902

Barbara Knebel
President
(W) 203/967-9767
(H) 203/967-8922
(FAX) 203/329-1358

Delaware

Maternal & Child Health -
Div of Public Health
Jesse Cooper Bldg
Federal & Water St
PO Box 637
Dover, DE 19903

Marihelen Barrett, RN, MSN
Director
(W) 302/739-4785

SIDS Info & Counseling Program -
Div Public Health
Federal & Water Streets
Cooper Building
Dover, DE 19903

Dennis Rubino, ACSW
Program Coordinator
(W) 302/739-4744

District Of Columbia

† Nation's Capitol Area Chapter
PO Box 3044
Oakton, VA 22124-3044

Deneena Herrera
President
Donna Shelton
Referral Coordinator
(W) 703/330-6241
(H) 703/435-7130
(SIDS #) 703/435-7130
(FAX) 703/759-4762

Maternal & Child Health Services
1660 L St, NW, Suite 904
Washington, DC 20036

Harry Lynch, MD
Director
(W) 202/673-6666

Commission of Public Health,
Div Comm Health Nursing
1905 East St SE
Washington, DC 20003

Mary Breach, RN, MSN
Nursing Coordinator
(W) 202/727-5122

Florida

† Southern Florida Chapter
12151 SW 51st Pl
Cooper City, FL 33330

Margie Simon
President
(W) 305/769-4700
(H) 305/680-9463
(FAX) 305/688-6215

† West Palm Beach Chapter
3802 Van Cott Circle
Lake Park, FL 33403

John Birney
President
Stephanie Quick
Referral Coordinator
(SIDS #) 407/624-8128
(H) 407/641-7126
(FAX) 407/747-2612

Central Florida Area Contact
4816 Cheval Blvd
Lutz, FL 33549

Marilyn Farber
Area Contact
(H) 813/949-2805

† Space Coast of Florida Chapter
481 Topeka Rd
Palm Bay, FL 32908

Helene Simon
President
(W) 407/725-1882

† Tampa Area Contact
11309 Loch Lomond Dr
Riverview, FL 33569

Suzanne Spiller
Area Contact
(H) 813/677-4374

Florida SIDS Program - Children's
1317 Winewood Blvd, Bldg 5,
State Health Office
Tallahassee, FL 32399-0700

Cynthia Studnic-Lewis, RN, MPH
Program Coordinator
(W) 904/488-2834

Div Maternal & Child Health -
Dept Health & Rehab
1323 Winewood Blvd, Bldg 1
Tallahassee, FL 32399-0700

Cynthia Studnic-Lewis, RN, MPH
Nursing Consultant
(W) 904/488-6005
(W) 904/487-1321

Georgia

Children's Health Services,
Georgia DHR
2600 Skyland Dr
Atlanta, GA 30319

Linette Jackson Hunt, MD, MPH
Director
(W) 404/320-0547

Div of Health Services -
Maternal & Child Health
878 Peachtree St, NE, Rm 217
Atlanta, GA 30309

Virginia Floyd, MD
Director
(W) 404/894-6622

Georgia Area Contact
305 C First Division
Fort Benning, GA 31905

Kathy D'Elousa
Area Contact
(H) 404/682-9970

† Atlanta Chapter
3415 Timbercreek Dr
Lawrenceville, GA 30093

Deb Baldwin
President
(W) 404/441-7626 X 3241
(H) 404/942-6820
(H) 404/564-2207
(SIDS #) 404/565-6333
  (outside GA)
(FAX) 404/448-7326

Hawaii

Hawaii SIDS Information &
Counseling Program
1319 Punahou St, 7th Fl Rm 739
Honolulu, HI 96826

Sharon Morton, RN
Nurse Consultant
(W) 808/947-8387
(H) 808/941-6155

Maternal & Child Health -
Hawaii Dept of Health
741-A Sunset Ave
Honolulu, HI 96816

Loretta Fuddy, ACSW, MPH
Acting Chief
(W) 808/737-8229

† Hawaii Chapter
1018 Iiwi St
Honolulu, HI 96816

Nancy Kern
President
(W) 808/548-2033
(H) 808/735-5125

Idaho

Bureau Maternal & Child Health,
ID Dept of Health
450 West State St
Boise, ID 83720

Simone deGlee
SIDS Coordinator
(W) 208/334-5957

† Idaho Area Contact
PO Box 831
Post Falls, ID 83854

Eileen Dickson
Area Contact
(H) 208/773-7981

Illinois

† Illinois SIDS Alliance
2320 Glenview Rd
Glenview, IL 60025

Joe Freveletti
Chairman
(W) 708/657-8080
(FAX) 708/657-7129
Karen Kohnke
Referral Coordinator
(W) 708/696-8776
(H) 708/894-8912
(H) 708/477-7481

† Peoria Branch of the Illinois
SIDS Alliance
PO Box 467
Hanna City, IL 61536

Kathy Dickinson
President
(W) 309/565-7144

† North Central Branch of the
Illinois SIDS Alliance
128 Split Oak Rd
Naperville, IL 60565

Georgia McDaniel
President
(W) 708/983-9254
(FAX) 708/357-6163

† Rockford Branch of the Illinois
SIDS Alliance
14771 Wittwer Rd
South Beloit, IL 61080

Tammy Tyrell
Area Contact
(H) 815/389-0966

Illinois SIDS Project
Dept of Public Health
535 West Jefferson St
Springfield, IL 62761

Lori Bennett
Chief Coordinator
Stephen Saunders, MD
(W) 217/785-4528

Indiana

† Northern Indiana SIDS Alliance
705 Studebaker
Mishawaka, IN 46544

Kathy Rosenthal
President
(W) 219/546-5464
(FAX) 219/297-1481

† Greater Indianapolis Chapter
5306 E 19th Pl
Indianapolis, IN 46218

Rick McKim
President
(W) 317/359-2534

SIDS Project Staff - IN State
Dept of Health
1330 W Michigan St, Rm 232-W
Indianapolis, IN 46205-1964

Larry Humbert
Chief Director
Judith Ganser, MD
(W) 317/633-8451
(W) 317/633-0722
(FAX) 317/633-0776

† West Central Lafayette Chapter
5934 Lookout Dr
West Lafayette, IN 47906

Jacqueline Bahler
President
(W) 317/447-6811 X 2810
(H) 317/567-2886

Iowa

† Illowa Guild for Infant Survival
PO Box 3586
Davenport, IA 52808

Melanie Pangburn
President
(W) 319/322-4870
(H) 319/323-1538
(FAX) 319/386-1321

Maternal & Child Health Bureau -
IA Dept of Health
Lucas State Office Building
Des Moines, IA 50319

Joyce Borgmeyer, MS
Chief
(W) 515/281-4911

Central Iowa Guild
PO Box 2274
Des Moines, IA 50310

Carol Thomas
President
(W) 515/278-5564
(FAX) 515/223-9301

Iowa SIDS Program - Iowa Dept
of Public Health
Lucas State Office Building
Des Moines, IA 50319

Janice Herndon
Director
(W) 515/281-4904
(H) 515/242-6384

Kansas

Northeastern Kansas Area Contact
1023 Elm St
Eudora, KS 66025

Cindy Higgins
Area Contact
(H) 913/542-2606

SIDS Resources - Kansas City
8430 Mission Rd, Suite 802
Shawnee Mission, KS 66206

Therese Kimberly
Director
(W) 913/649-6996

KS Dept of Health & Environment -
Maternal & Child Health
900 SW Jackson St, 10th Fl
Topeka, KS 66612-1290

Azzie Young, PhD
Acting Director
(W) 913/296-1300

† Kansas Chapter
4408 N Edgmoor
Wichita, KS 67220

Mary Luebbert
President
(H) 316/744-9955

Kentucky

† Tri-State SIDS Chapter
6009 Dee Ct
Ashland, KY 41102

Deena Williams
President
(SIDS #) 606/928-3459

† Northern Kentucky/Greater
Cincinnati Chapter
Childrens Medical Center, CH 5-20
240 Bethesda Ave
Cincinnati, OH 45229

Beverly Stewart
President
(H) 606/261-6736
(FAX) 606/344-3968
Attn: Marketing

Information & Counseling
Program - KY DHR
275 E Main St
Frankfort, KY 40621-0001

Ida Lyons, RN
Program Coordinator
(W) 502/564-3236

† Kentucky Chapter
PO Box 22085
Louisville, KY 40252-0085

Marie McBrearty
President
(W) 502/245-7068
(FAX) 606/277-1832

Louisiana

SIDS Info & Counseling Program -
  Maternal & Child Health
PO Box 60630
New Orleans, LA 70160

Joan Wightkin, MPH
Administrator
Jamie Roques, RNC
SIDS Coordinator
(W) 504/568-5073

† Central Louisiana Area Contact
  124 Alice Dr
  Pineville, LA 71360

Donna Street
Area Contact
(H) 318/448-4233

Maine

† Maine Chapter
  118 Wardtown Rd
  Freeport, ME 04210

Robert McConnell
President
(H) 207/865-1825
(FAX) 207/865-0212

Maine SIDS Program - Maine Dept
  Human Resources
151 Capitol St,
  Statehouse, Station 11
Augusta, ME 04333-0011

Eleanor Bruce, RN, MEd
Director
Kathleen Jewett
Program Coordinator
(W) 207/289-3259

Maryland

Maryland SIDS Info & Counseling
  Project UMAB
WP Carter Center
630 W Fayette St, Rm 5-684
Baltimore, MD 21201

Daniel Timmel, MSW
Project Director
(W) 410/328-5062
(H) 410/945-6044
(FAX) 410/328-8742

Office of Infant, Child &
  Adolescent Health Service
Dept of Health & Mental Hygiene
201 W Preston St, Rm 321A
Baltimore, MD 21201

Polly Harrison, MD
Chief
(W) 410/225-6749

† Sudden Infant Death Syndrome
  Alliance, Inc
10500 Little Patuxent Parkway,
Suite 420
Columbia, MD 21044

Robert Hinnen
Coordinator
Thomas L. Moran
President
(W) 410/964-8000
(SIDS #) 800/221-7437

Massachusetts

Maternal & Child Health - MA Dept
Public Health
150 Tremont St
Boston, MA 02111

Deborah Klein Walker, EdD
Director
(W) 617/727-3372

Massachusetts Center for SIDS -
Boston City Hospital
818 Harrison Ave
Boston, MA 02118

Mary McClain, RN, MS
Project Coordinator
(W) 617/534-5742
(SIDS #) 617/534-7437
(FAX) 617/534-5555

† Massachusetts Chapter
91 Parker View St
Springfield, MA 01129

Penny Begley
President
(W) 413/783-7459

Michigan

Michigan State SIDS Center
1200 6th St, 9th Flr
North Tower
Detroit, MI 48226

Gina Schaffer
Program Coordinator
(W) 313/256-2153
(H) 313/522-3668
800/359-3722
(FAX) 313/236-1844

† Grand Rapids Area Chapter
PO Box 9323
Grand Rapids, MI 45909-0323

Gail Lilly
President
(W) 616/364-8766
(H) 616/534-6641
(FAX) 616/774-3884

Grand Rapids SIDS Program
700 Fuller NE
Grand Rapids, MI 49503

Colleen Jillson, RN
Coordinator
(W) 616/774-3040

† Southeastern Michigan Chapter
2158 Lennox
Grosse Pointe Woods, MI 48236

Terry Schaffer
President
Laura Reno
Referral Coordinator
(W) 313/884-4742
(W) 312/652-8253

Maternal & Child Health - Dept
of Public Health
3423 N Logan St
Lansing, MI 48909

Cheryl Lauber, MSN
SIDS Chief Lead
Ronald Uken
Acting Director
(W) 517/335-8989
(W) 517/335-8955
(FAX) 517/335-9491

† West Shore of Michigan Chapter
Route 1, Box 151
Montague, MI 49437

Terry Smith
President
(H) 616/894-9596

Macomb County Health Department
43525 Elizabeth Rd
Mt Clemens, MI 48053

Loretta Lindsay, RN
Coordinator
(W) 313/469-5520

Michigan Area Contact
Marquette County Health
Department
184 US 41 West
Negaunee, MI 49866

Connie Rhoades, RN
Area Contact
(W) 906/475-9312

Oakland County Health Division
1200 North Telegraph
Pontiac, MI 48053

Peggy Conrad, PHN
SIDS Coordinator
(W) 313/858-1379

† North Central/Southwestern
Michigan Chapter
5241 Windy Ridge
Portage, MI 49001

Doug Harris
President
(W) 616/384-9338
(H) 616/345-4309

Minnesota

Maternal & Child Health -
Dept of Health
717 Delaware SE, PO Box 9441
Minneapolis, MN 55440

Carolyn McKay, MD, MPH
Director
(W) 612/623-5166

Minnesota Sudden Infant
Death Center
2525 Chicago Ave, South
Minneapolis, MN 55404

Kathleen Fernbach, PHN
Project Coordinator
(W) 612/863-6285
(SIDS #) 800/732-3812 (in MN)
(FAX) 612/863-6912

Mississippi

SIDS Info & Counseling Program -
Child Health Services
PO Box 1700
Jackson, MS 39215-1700

Geneva Cannon, MS, MPH
Nurse Consultant
(W) 601/960-7441

Bureau of Health Services -
MS Dept of Health
2423 N State St
Jackson, MS 39215-1700

Terry Beck, MSW
Chief
(W) 601/960-7463

Missouri

Maternal, Child & Family
Health, MO Dept of Health
PO Box 570
Jefferson City, MO 65102

Lorna Wilson, RN, MSPH
Director
(W) 314/751-6174

SIDS Resources - Missouri
Division of Health
PO Box 570
Jefferson City, MO 65102

Connie Cunningham
Service Coordinator
(W) 314/751-6215

SIDS Resources - Kansas City
8430 Mission Rd, Suite 802
Shawnee Mission, KS 66206

Therese Kimberly
Director
(W) 913/649-6996

SIDS Resources, Inc
929 DeMun Ave
St Louis, MO 63105

Helen Fuller, MSW
Executive Director
(W) 314/862-3033
(SIDS #) 800/421-3511
(in MO only)
(FAX) 314/862-3822

Montana

Montana Dept of Health
Div of Health Services &
MCH Bureau
Cogswell Bldg
Helena, MT 59620

Maxine Ferguson, RN, MN
Chief
(W) 406/444-4740

† Montana SIDS Alliance
PO Box 3294
Missoula, MT 59806

Rick Johns
President
(W) 406/251-3600
(H) 406/273-6559

Nebraska

Maternal & Child Health -
Department of Health
301 Centennial Mall South -
3rd Fl, PO Box 95007
Lincoln, NE 68509-5007

David P. Schor, MD, FAAP
Director
(W) 402/471-0784

Nebraska SIDS Foundation
600 S 42nd St
Omaha, NE 68198-2106

Fran Farris
President
Karen Kleine
Referral Coordinator
(W) 402/559-7317

Nevada

Maternal & Child Health -
State DHR
505 E King St, Rm 205
Carson City, NV 89710

Yvonne Wimett, BS, MPA
Manager
(W) 702/687-4885

† Nevada Clark County Chapter
651 Shadow Ln
Las Vegas, NV 89106

Mary K Pedersen-Hernandez
Coordinator
(W) 702/455-4344 or 4103
(H) 702/368-2976

New Hampshire

NH SIDS Program - Maternal
& Child Health Bureau
6 Hazen Dr - Human Services Bldg
Concord, NH 03301-6527

Charles Albano
Chief
(W) 603/271-4596
Audrey Knight, MSN, CPNP
SIDS Coordinator
(W) 603/271-4536
800/852-3345 (in NH)
(FAX) 603/271-3745

† Southern New Hampshire/
NASHUA
Area Chapter
45 Lawrence St
Pepperell, MA 01463

Ron Koivu
President
(W) 508/433-2383

New Jersey

† New Jersey Chapter
  100 Jersey Ave, Bldg D7
  New Brunswick, NJ 08901

Susan Champa
President
(W) 908/548-7251
(SIDS #) 609/890-8008
(FAX) 908/780-6886

New Jersey SIDS Resource Center
254 Easton Ave
New Brunswick, NJ 08903

Tara Ryan
Coordinator
(W) 201/249-2160
(SIDS #) 800/545-7437 (in NJ)
(FAX) 908/249-6306

Parental & Child Health
  Service - NJ Dept of Health
363 W State St - CN 364
Trenton, NJ 08625-0364

George Halpin, MD
Director
(W) 609/292-5656
Judith Hall
Hlth Care Svcs Eval
(W) 609/292-5616

New Mexico

SIDS Info & Counseling
  Program - Medical Invest Ofc
University of New Mexico
School of Medicine
Albuquerque, NM 87131

Beverly White, RN, MS
Director
(W) 505/277-3053
(H) 505/296-4125
(FAX) 505/277-0727

† New Mexico Chapter
  13106 Cedarbrook, NE
  (PO Box 40577)
  Albuquerque, NM 87197-0577

Kari Bradenburg
President
(W) 505/842-5924
(H) 505/296-9576

Maternal & Child Health - Dept
  of Health & Environment
PO Box 968
Santa Fe, NM 87504-0968

Ann Taulbee, MBA
Chief
(W) 505/827-2350

New York

NY State Dept of Health -
  Child & Adolescent Health Bureau
Corning Tower Bldg,
  Empire State Plaza, Rm 780
Albany, NY 12237

Monica Meyer, MD
Director
(W) 518/474-7922

† Western New York Chapter
3580 Harlem Rd, Suite 5
Buffalo, NY 14215

Karen Koster
President
(H) 716/649-7272
Mary Ellen Flynn
Executive Director
(SIDS#) 716/837-7438
(W) 716/837-7438

† Long Island Chapter
PO Box 342
Deer Park, NY 11729

Chris Bayliss
President
(H) 516/399-2070
(SIDS #) 516/321-7437

Western New York SIDS Center
200 Fairport Village Landing
Fairport, NY 14450

M. Gabrielle Weiss, BPS
Director
(W) 716/223-5110

NY City Info & Counseling
Program for SIDS
Medical Examiner's Office
520 First Ave, Rm 506
New York, NY 10016

Judith Gaines, CSW, PhD
Program Director
(W) 212/686-8854
(FAX) 212/447-2716

† Genesee Valley Chapter
PO Box 17424
Rochester, NY 14617

Dan Weatherly
President
(W) 716/724-7148
(H) 716/889-4512
(SIDS #) 716/223-1888

† Hudson-Mohawk Chapter
2431 Barton Ave
Rotterdam, NY 12306

Frank LeGere
President
(W) 518/355-5984
(FAX) 518/459-1038

† Syracuse Chapter
1409 Grant Blvd
Syracuse, NY 13208

Nessa Vercillo-Degirolamo
(SIDS #) 315/474-1656
(FAX) 315/478-0204

Eastern New York State SIDS
Regional Center
School of Social Welfare,
State University of New York
Stony Brook, NY 11794-8232

Marie Chandick, CSW
Director
(W) 516/444-3690
(FAX) 516/444-7565

North Carolina

† North Carolina - Greater
   Piedmont Chapter
4970 Weddington Rd
Concord, NC 28027

Brenda Hatley
President
(H) 704/782-2353

NC SIDS Info & Counseling
   Program - Maternal & Child Health
Dept of Environmental Health
PO Box 27687
Raleigh, NC 27611-7687

Ann Wolf, MD
Director
(W) 919/733-3816
Dianne Tyson, BSW
Program Assistant
(W) 919/733-7791
(FAX) 919/733-0488

† Winston-Salem Area Contact
4664 Old Belews Creek Rd
Winston-Salem, NC 27101

Terry Spangler
Contact
(SIDS #) 919/723-5711

North Dakota

† North Dakota Chapter
128 Apollo Ave
Bismarck, ND 58501

Barb Delvo
President
(W) 701/255-3090
(H) 701/224-1600
(SIDS #) 701/667-2006
(FAX) 216/379-8152

ND Dept of Health Program -
   Maternal & Child Health Div
Village of Family Services
308 Second Ave SW
Minot, ND 58701

Sue Saltsman, RN
Coordinator
(W) 701/857-7695

Ohio

† North Eastern Ohio Chapter -
   Childrens Hospital
Medical Center of Akron
281 Locust St
Akron, OH 43708

Linda Hardman
President
(W) 800/537-4105
(H) 216/397-0839
(FAX) 216/379-8152
Pat Marquis
Director
(W) 216/379-8915
(FAX) 216/379-8152

† Greater Cincinnati Chapter/
    Northern Kentucky
College of Medicine, Rm 6133
240 Bethesda Ave
Cincinnati, OH 45229-2899

Beverly Stewart, RN
President
(W) 606/261-6736
(FAX) 606/344-3968

Cleveland Support Group -
    Rainbow Babies Hospital
2074 Abbington Rd
Cleveland, OH 44106

Susan Koziol, RN
Director
(SIDS #) 216/844-1301

OH SIDS Info & Counseling
Dept of Health
Maternal & Child Health Bureau
246 N High St, PO Box 118
Columbus, OH 43266-0118

James Quilty, MD
Chief
(W) 614/466-3263
Ben Chukwumah, MD, MPH
Project Director
(W) 614/466-4716
(FAX) 614/644-9850

† Central Ohio Chapter
1816 Kent St
Columbus, OH 43205

Brent Porter
President
(SIDS #) 614/252-8135
(OH only) 800/421-1633

Elyria Support Group
c/o Lisa Sellers
303 Eastern Heights Blvd
Elyria, OH 44035

Lisa Sellers
Area Contact
(H) 612/988-7274

† Northwest Ohio Chapter
13105 Weuroth Highway
Jasper, MI 49248

Melanie Wyse
President
(W) 517/443-5736

Marion Support Group
1107 Martinique
Marion, OH 43302

Sherry Snyder
President
(W) 614/387-3528

† Miami Valley Chapter
8222 E New Carlisle Rd
New Carlisle, OH 45344

Thomas Bono
President
(SIDS #) 513/845-9180
(FAX) 513/845-9765

New Philadelphia Support Group
1625 Rolland Ave, NE
New Philadelphia, OH 44663

Barbara Airgood
(W) 216/343-5833

Southeast Ohio Support Group
980 Main St
Sciotoville, OH

Johnita Ramsey
(H) 614/776-7673
(W) 614/353-4330

Oklahoma

Maternal & Child Health -
State Dept of Health
1000 NE Tenth St, Rm 703
Oklahoma City, OK 73117-1299

Sara Reed DePersio, MD, MPH
Medical Director
(W) 405/271-4471

† Oklahoma Chapter
7829 S Young
Oklahoma City, OK 73159

Sharon Matthews
President
(H) 405/686-1322

Oklahoma SIDS Program
Oklahoma State Health Department
Oklahoma City, OK 73159

Ronna Vaughn
Coordinator
(W) 405/271-4471
(FAX) 405/271-6199

Oregon

† Oregon Chapter
PO Box 1641
Beaverton, OR 97075-1641

Marjorie Ehlen
President
Wendy Patterson
Referral Coordinator
(Chapter) 503/643-1470
(W) 206/254-7936
(H) 503/244-2243

Office of Health Services -
OR State Health Division
1400 SW 5th Ave, Rm 508
Portland, OR 97207

Donna Clark, RN
Assistant Administrator
(W) 503/229-6380

SIDS Info & Counseling Program -
Maternal & Child Health
Program
1400 SW Fifth Ave (PO Box 231)
Portland, OR 97207

Sue Omel, RN, MPH
Child Health Coordinator
(W) 503/229-6617

Pennsylvania

Maternal & Child Health -
PA Dept of Health
PO Box 90, Rm 725
Health & Welfare Bldg
Harrisburg, PA 17108

Evelyn Bouden, MD
Director
(W) 717/787-7443

Pennsylvania SIDS Center -
Philadelphia
834 Chestnut St #200
Benjamin Franklin House
Philadelphia, PA 19107

Rosanne English, RN
Executive Director
(W) 215/955-1400
(SIDS #) 800/258-7434 (in PA)
(FAX) 215/923-2989

† Philadelphia Area Chapter
PO Box 8206
Philadelphia, PA 19101

Chester Slye
President
(W) 215/722-7437
(FAX) 215/874-7775

† Western Pennsylvania Chapter
SIDS Office
South Side Hospital
2000 Mary St
Pittsburgh, PA 15203

Judy Bannon
Executive Director
Chuck Puskar
Chairman
(SIDS #) 412/481-1410
(W) 412/481-1410
(FAX) 412/481-5968

Puerto Rico

Maternal & Child Health -
Department of Health
Commonwealth of Puerto Rico
Call Box 70184
San Juan, PR 00936

Rafael Varela, MD, MPH
Director
(W) 809/754-9580

Rhode Island

RI Dept of Health - Family Health
& Crippled Children's Svs
SID Info & Counseling
3 Capitol Hill, Rm 302
Providence, RI 02908

William Hollingshead, MD
Chief
(W) 401/277-2312
Anne M. Roache, RN
SIDS Coordinator
(W) 401/277-2312

† Rhode Island Chapter
377 Spring Green Rd
Warwick, RI 02888

Mary Wilks
President
(SIDS #) 401/463-7050

South Carolina

Maternal & Child Health -
  SC Dept Health & Environment
2600 Bull St
Columbia, SC 29201

Sara E. Bulcerek, MSN, CMN
Director
(W) 803/737-4000

SIDS Info & Counseling -
  SC Dept Health & Environment
2600 Bull St
Columbia, SC 29201

Brenda Cresswell, ACSW, LMSW
SIDS Coordinator
(SIDS #) 803/737-4079

South Dakota

SIDS Info Program -
  SD Dept of Health
Public Safety Building
118 W Capitol St
Pierre, SD 57501

Sandra Durick, BA
Director
(W) 605/773-3737

Tennessee

SIDS/APNEA Center - Memphis
Baptist Memorial Hospital
899 Madison Ave
Memphis, TN 38146

Mary Beth Troy
Coordinator
(SIDS #) 901/766-5808

† Middle Tennessee Chapter
PO Box 110361
Nashville, TN 37222-0361

Beverly Peery
President
(W) 615/895-9545

TN Dept of Health
Tennessee SIDS Program -
  Maternal & Child Health
525 Cordell Hull Bldg
Nashville, TN 37247-4701

Judith Womack, RN
Director
(W) 615/741-7353

Texas

† Greater Tarrant County/
  Ft Worth Chapter
Route 4, Box 902
Alvarado, TX 76009

Janice James
President
(H) 817/783-3850

Area Contact
4325 Omaha
Amarillo, TX 79106

Pat Bartlett
Area Contact
(H) 806/355-1548

† Austin Area Chapter
PO Box 16674
Austin, TX 78761

Mary Anne Schmidt
President
(W) 512/499-7040
(SIDS #) 512/473-6900

TX SIDS Info & Counseling -
Maternal & Child Health
1100 West 49th St
Austin, TX 78756

Linda Prentice, MD
Program Coordinator
(W) 512/458-7700

North Texas SIDS Info &
Counseling Program
PO Box 35728
Dallas, TX 75235

Leslie Malone, MS
Project Coordinator
(W) 214/688-2786

† Dallas Chapter
5213 Baker
The Colony, TX 75116

Donna & David Parkhill
President
(H) 214/370-3250
(W) 214/385-0680

Harris County SIDS Info &
Counseling Program
2501 Dunstan, PO Box 25249
Houston, TX 77265

Kathleen Ingrando, RN, BSN
Program Coordinator
(SIDS #) 713/620-6895

† Greater Houston Chapter
5714 Cerritos Rd
Houston, TX 77035

Sharon Endelman
President
Laura Bennett
Referral Coordinator
(H) 713/728-0679
(W) 713/937-0679
(SIDS #) 713/937-9819
(FAX) 713/342-3743

Southwest SIDS Research Institute
Brazosport Memorial Hospital
100 Medical Dr
Lake Jackson, TX 77566

Judy Henslee
Coordinator
(W) 409/297-4411 1814
(SIDS #) 800/245-7437
(FAX) 409/297-6905

Texas Area Contact
5215 91st
Lubbock, TX

Robert Freeman, MD
Area Contact
(H) 806/794-6940

Area Contact
1310 Chapter
San Angelo, TX 76901

Judy Summersgill
Area Contact
(H) 915/655-9064

† San Antonio Chapter
9814 Autumn Star
San Antonio, TX 78250-5801

Robyn O'Neal
President
(W) 512/925-2971
(H) 512/680-4843

† North Texas/Southern Oklahoma
    Chapter
35 A Nehls
Shepherd AFB, TX 76311

Lisa Sommers
President
(SIDS #) 817/855-4420
(FAX) 817/761-8348

Utah

† Utah Chapter
2881 W 4450 South
Roy, UT 84067

Jeff Hannes
President
(W) 801/250-7618

Utah SIDS Program -
  Health Services Dept
Bureau of Child Health
PO Box 16650
288 N 1460 West
Salt Lake City, UT 84116-0650

Kathleen Glasheen, RN, MS
Director
Karen Nash, RN, MS, PNP
Program Coordinator
(W) 801/538-6140

Vermont

Vermont SIDS Program - Dept
  of Health, Medical Services
PO Box 70, 1193 North Ave
Burlington, VT 05402

Cindy Ingham, RN, BSN
Director
(W) 802/863-7333

Virgin Islands

Department of Health
Charlotte Amalie
St Thomas, VI 00802

Alfred O. Heath, MD
Commissioner
(W) 809/776-3580

Virginia

† Nation's Capitol Area Chapter
PO Box 3044
Oakton, VA 22124-3044

Deneena Hererra
President
Donna Shelton
Referral Coordinator
(W) 703/330-6241
(W) 703/435-7130
(SIDS #) 703/435-7130
(FAX) 703/759-4762

Virginia SIDS Program -
    Maternal & Child Health
Dept of Health
109 Governor St
Richmond, VA 23219

Alice Linyear, MD
Director
(W) 804/786-7367
Arlethia Rogers, RN
Nurse Consultant

Virginia Beach/Norfolk American
    Guild for Infant Survival, Inc
1565 Laskin Rd
Virginia Beach, VA 23451

Scott & Eileen Hessek
(H) 804/463-3845
(FAX) 804/491-8812

Washington

Parent & Child Health Services
Maternal Health Service
Airdustrial Park Bldg #3,
    MS, LC-12A
Olympia, WA 98504

Fran Moellman
Program Manager
(W) 206/752-2482

Parent & Child Health Services
Dept of Health
Mail Stop LC-11A
Olympia, WA 98504

Maxine Hayes, MD, MPH
Director
(W) 206/753-7021

Thurston County SIDS Guild
1023 SE Adams, #287
Olympia, WA 98501

Andrea Damatio
President
(W) 206/923-1231
(SIDS #) 206/923-1225
(FAX) 206/923-1231

† Washington State Chapter
c/o Children's Hospital &
  Medical Center
4800 Sand Point Way, NE
Seattle, WA 98105

Richard Beszhak
President
Nancy Freeman
Executive Director
(W) 206/999-0496
(W) 206/526-2110
(H) 206/821-8380
(FAX) 206/226-5779

SIDS Northwest Regional Center
Childrens Hospital
4800 Sand Point Way, NE
PO Box C-5371
Seattle, WA 98105

Lauren Valk Lawson, MN
Director
(W) 206/526-2100

† Eastern Washington Branch Office
W 508 - Sixth, Suite B
Spokane, WA 99204

Carol Moore
President
Bev Younglund
Parent Contact
(W) 509/456-0505

West Virginia

† Tri-State SIDS Chapter
6009 Dee Ct
Ashland, KY 41102

Deena Williams
President
(SIDS #) 606/928-3459

West Virginia SIDS Program
WV Health Department
1411 Virginia St, East
Charleston, WV 25301

Joan R. Kenney, RN
Director
(W) 304/348-5388

WV SIDS Project
Department of Pediatrics
West Virginia University
Room 4621 Basic Science Bldg
Morgantown, WV 26505

David Myerberg, MD
Director
(W) 304/348-8870

Wisconsin

Department of Health &
  Social Services
1414 E Washington Ave, Rm 96
Madison, WI 53703-3044

Richard Aaronson
Director
(W) 608/266-2003

Wisconsin Div of Health
Dept Health/Social Services
One W Wilson St, PO Box 309
Madison, WI 53701-0309

Murray Katcher, MD, PhD
Chief
(W) 608/266-9823

SIDS Counseling & Research Ctr
9000 W Wisconsin Ave
PO Box 1997
Milwaukee, WI 53201

Kathy Geracie, BSW
Program Coordinator
(SIDS #) 414/266-2743

Wyoming

Div of Health/Medical Svcs
WY Dept of Health
Hathaway Bldg
Cheyenne, WY 82002-0710

J. Richard Hillman, MD, PhD
Administrator
(W) 307/777-6186

† Wyoming Chapter
4714 E 17th St
Cheyenne, WY 82001

Jennifer Poteet
President
(SIDS #) 307/632-7609

ADDITIONAL RESOURCES

Council of Guilds for
   Infant Survival
8178 Nadine River Circle
Fountain Valley, CA 92708

Chris Elliott
President
800/247-4370
(FAX) 714/834-8741
c/o Penny Stastny

American Academy of Pediatrics
141 Northwest Point Blvd
Elk Grove Village, IL 60009

708/228-5005

The Compassionate Friends, Inc
National Office
PO Box 3696
Oak Brook, IL 60522-3696

Therese Goodrich
Director
708/990-0010

Pregnancy and Infant Loss Support
SHARE National Headquarters
(Source of Help in Airing &
   Resolving Experiences)
St Josephs Health Center
300 First Capitol Dr
St Charles, MO 63301

Cathi Lammert
Director
314/947-5000

Association of SIDS Program   Mary McClain, RN
  Professionals   President
Massachusetts Center for SIDS   617/534-7437
Boston City Hospital
818 Harrison Ave
Boston, MA 02118

Pregnancy and Infant Loss Center   Sherokee Ilse
1415 E Wayzata Blvd, Suite 105   Director
Wayzata, MN 55391   612/473-9372

National SIDS Resource Center   Saranne Booth
8201 Greensboro Dr, Suite 600   Executive Director
McLean, VA 22102   703/821-8955
                                     (FAX) 703/506-0384

Sudden Infant Death Syndrome   Thomas L. Moran
  Alliance   President
10500 Little Patuxent Pkwy   800/221-7437
Suite 420   (24-hr hotline)
Columbia, MD 21044

Apnea Identification Program   Karen Braniff, RN, CNS
3901 Beaubian   313/745-4301
Detroit, MI 48201

Humanistic Foundation's   800/333-4444
Suicide Prevention Hotline

Consumer Product Safety   General Specialist
  Commission   301/504-0580
OIPA Department
5401 W Bard Ave
Bethesda, MD 20207

SIDS International

National SIDS Council for Australia Karen Fitzgerald
1227 Malvern Rd   (W) 61-3-822-7022
Malvern, Victoria 3144   (FAX) 61-3-822-7603
AUSTRALIA

GEPS   Dr Christa Einspieler
Department of Physiology   (W) 43-316/380-4276
University Graz   (FAX) 43-316/38-3686
Harrachgasse 21/5
A-8010 GRAZ
AUSTRIA

Naatschappelijki Zetel SIDS vzw   Bert Gysel
Koerspleindreef 48
2950 Kalpellen
BELGIUM

Canadian Foundation for the   Beverley De Bruyn
  Study of Infant Death   Executive Director
PO Box 190 Station R   (W) 416/488-3260
Toronto, Ontario M4G 3Z9   (FAX) 416/488-3864
CANADA

MuDr Jiri Jura   . . .
02S - detska amb
013 06 Terchova
CZECHOSLOVAKIA

IV detska klinika   Dr Hana Houstkova
Ke Karlovu   Dr Jiri Zewan
120 00 Praha 2
CZECHOSLOVAKIA

Agrupaciom de Padres Para La   . . .
  Prevencion del Syndrome Infantile
  de Muerte Subita Muestra Sauroa
  de Los Angeles 116
El Golf
Santiago
CHILE

Foraeldre og Foedsel   Orla Kristensen
Bag Moellen 6   .   (W) 45-42-612750
276-Greve   (FAX) 45-33-158600
DENMARK

The Foundation for the   June Reed
  Study of Infant Deaths   (W) 071-235-0965
35 Belgrave Square   (FAX) 071-823-1986
London SW1X 8QB
ENGLAND

Naitre et Vivra   Dominique Van Belle
71 Rue Notre Dame des Champs   (W) 1-4633-0260
75006 Paris   (FAX) 1-4046-8491
FRANCE

GEPS
Postfach 610149
D-7000
Stuttgart 61
WEST GERMANY

Frau Susan Juptner

Foundation of Research
  in Childhood
42 Amalias St
Athens 10558
GREECE

Meropi Michaleli

Department of Forensic Medicine
Semmelweis University
  Medical School
H-1450 Budapest, Pf 9/41
HUNGARY

Dr Eva Keller

Irish SIDS Association
Carmichael House
4 North Brunswick St
Dublin 7
IRELAND

Eimear Berry

Associazione Italiana SIDS
Via Giovanni Mayr
10-20122 Milan
ITALY

Signora Alessandra
Campisi Garbagnati

Nagoya City University
  Medical School
Kawasumi, Mizuho, Nagoya
JAPAN

Dr Hajime Togari
Chief, Neonatology
Associate Professor
Pediatrics

National Children's
  Health Foundation
PO Box 28-177
Auckland 5
NEW ZEALAND

Dr Shirley Tonkin
(W) 64-9-524-8597
(FAX) 64-9-524-8466

Lands Forenigen til stotte
  ved krybbedod
Postboks 97
Ulleval Sykehus
0407 Oslo 4
NORWAY

Norwegian SIDS Society
Arbinsgate 7
0253 Oslo
NORWAY

Jorun Eggen
(W) 47-2-437680
(FAX) 47-2-438920

Lung Function Unit
Centrum Zdrowia Dziecka
  Pomnik-Szpital
Dzial Diagnostycany
Aleja Dzieci Polskich 20
04-736 Warszawa - Miedzylesie
POLAND

Dr P. Gutkowski

Instituto de Medicina Legal
  de Lisboa
Rua Manuel Bento de Sousa No 3
1100 Lisboa
PORTUGAL

Ms Isabel Pinto Ribeiro

Scottish Cot Death Trust
Royal Hospital for Sick Children
Yorkhill
Glasgow G3 8SJ
SCOTLAND

Hazel Brooke
(W) 041-357-3946
(FAX) 041-334-1376

Cot Death Foundation (RSA)
34 Julia St
Birchleigh North
Kempton Park 1619
SOUTH AFRICA

Anne Lehmkuhl

The Swedish SIDS Parent Group
Jamtbovagen 2
Garpenberg 77073
SWEDEN

Asa Ljunggren
(W) 46-225-20570
(FAX) 46-879-23902

GEPS Institute fur Anatomie
  der Universitat Zurich - Irchel
Winterhurer Strasse 190
8057 Zurich
SWITZERLAND

Frau Prof Dr G. Molz

Foundation for the Parents of
  Cot Death Children
Postbus 293
6700 AG Wageningen
THE NETHERLANDS

Nel & Dirk Werdekken
(W) 033-751487

Institute of Pediatrics
Academy of Medical Sciences
Lomousovskij np 2
Moscow
USSR

Professor V. Tatochenko

Department of Pediatrics No 3
Leningrad Pediatric Medical
Institute
Litovskaya 2
Lenningrad, 194 100
USSR

Professor Vorontsov

National SIDS Foundation
of Zimbabwe
5 Kimloch Ave
North End
Byulawayo
ZIMBABWE

. . .

APPENDIX P

THE MEDICAL HOME

The American Academy of Pediatrics believes that the medical care of infants, children, and adolescents ideally should be accessible, continuous, comprehensive, family centered, coordinated, and compassionate. It should be delivered or directed by well-trained physicians who are able to manage or facilitate essentially all aspects of pediatric care. The physician should be known to the child and family and should be able to develop a relationship of mutual responsibility and trust with them. These characteristics define the "medical home" and describe the care that has traditionally been provided by pediatricians in an office setting. In contrast, care provided through emergency rooms, walk-in clinics, and other urgent care facilities is often less effective and more costly.

We should strive to attain a "medical home" for all of our children. While geographic barriers, manpower constraints, practice patterns, and economic and social forces make the ideal "medical home" unobtainable for many children, we believe that comprehensive health care of infants, children, and adolescents, wherever delivered, should encompass the following services:

1. Provision of preventive care including, but not restricted to, immunizations, growth and development assessments, appropriate screening, health care supervision, and patient and parental counselling about health and psychosocial issues.

2. Assurance of ambulatory and inpatient care for acute illnesses, 24 hours a day, 7 days a week; during the working day, after hours, on weekends, 52 weeks of the year.

3. Provision of care over an extended period of time to enhance continuity.

4. Identification of the need for subspecialty consultation and referrals and knowing from whom and where these can be obtained. Provision of medical information about the patient to the consultant. Evaluation of the consultant's recommendations, implementation of recommendations that are indicated and appropriate, and interpretation of these to the family.

5. Interaction with school and community agencies to be certain that special health needs of the individual child are addressed.

6. Maintenance of a central record and data base containing all pertinent medical information about the child, including information about hospitalizations. This record should be accessible, but confidentiality must be assured.

Medical care of infants, children, and adolescents must sometimes be provided in locations other than physicians' offices. However, unless these locations provide all of the services listed above, they do not meet the definition of a medical home. Other venues for children's care include hospital outpatient clinics, school-based and school-linked clinics, community health centers, health department clinics, and others. However, wherever given, medical care coverage must be constantly available. It should be supervised by physicians well trained in primary pediatric medicine, preferably pediatricians. Whenever possible, the physician should be physically present where the care is provided; but it may be necessary for the physician to direct other health care providers such as nurses, nurse practitioners, and physician assistants off site. Whether physically present or not, the physician must act as the child's advocate and assume control and ultimate responsibility for the care that is provided.

Michael D. Dickens, MD, FAAP
John L. Green, MD, FAAP
Alan E. Kohrt, MD, FAAP
Howard A. Pearson, MD, FAAP
Ad Hoc Task Force on Definition of the Medical Home

APPENDIX Q

**Model Legislation
SENATE, No. 408**

**STATE OF NEW JERSEY
INTRODUCED FEBRUARY 24, 1992**

**By Senators CAFIERO, BROWN
AND DiFRANCESCO**

AN ACT concerning emergency medical services for children and supplementing chapter 2K of Title 26 of the Revised Statutes.

BE IT ENACTED by the Senate and General Assembly of the State of New Jersey:

1. The Legislature finds and declares that:

   a. Traumatic injuries, such as automobile accidents, bicycle accidents, drownings and poisonings, are the most common cause of death in children over the age of one; and children have a high death rate in these emergency situations.

   b. Children react differently than adults to stress, metabolize drugs differently, and suffer different illnesses and injuries. Because of these differences, children's emergency medical needs should be recognized.

   c. Emergency medical services training programs focus on adults and, therefore, offer fewer hours of pediatric training. In addition, many emergency medical services personnel have no clinical experience with children, indicating the need to improve training of these personnel in pediatric emergencies.

d. It is the public policy of this State that children are entitled to comprehensive emergency medical services, including prehospital, hospital and rehabilitative care.

2. As used in this act:

"Advanced life support" means an advanced level of prehospital, interhospital, and emergency service care which includes basic life support functions, cardiac monitoring, cardiac defibrillation, telemetered electrocardiography, administration of antiarrhythmic agents, intravenous therapy, administration of specific medications, drugs and solutions, use of adjunctive ventilation devices, trauma care and other techniques and procedures authorized in writing by the commissioner pursuant to department regulations and P.L. 1984, c.146 (C.26:2K-7 et seq.).

"Advisory council" means the Emergency Medical Services for Children Advisory Council established pursuant to section 5 of this act.

"Basic life support" means a basic level of prehospital care which includes patient stabilization, airway clearance, cardiopulmonary resuscitation, hemorrhage control, initial wound care and fracture stabilization, and other techniques and procedures authorized by the commissioner.

"Commissioner" means the Commissioner of Health.

"Coordinator" means the person coordinating the EMSC program within the Office of Emergency Medical Services in the Department of Health.

"Department" means the Department of Health.

"EMSC program" means the Emergency Medical Services for Children program established pursuant to section 3 of this act, and other relevant programmatic activities conducted by the Office of Emergency Medical Services in the Department of Health in support of appropriate treatment, transport, and triage of ill or injured children in New Jersey.

"Emergency medical services personnel" means persons trained and certified or licensed to provide emergency medical care, whether on a paid or volunteer basis, as part of a basic life support or advanced life support prehospital emergency care service or in an emergency department or pediatric critical care or specialty unit in a licensed hospital.

"Prehospital care" means the provision of emergency medical care or transportation by trained and certified or licensed emergency medical services personnel at the scene of an emergency and while transporting sick or injured persons to a medical care facility or provider.

3. a. There is established within the Office of Emergency Medical Services in the Department of Health, the Emergency Medical Services for Children program.

   b. The commissioner shall hire a full-time coordinator for the EMSC program in consultation with, and by the recommendation of the advisory council.

   c. The coordinator shall implement the EMSC program following consultation with, and at the recommendation of, the advisory council. The coordinator shall serve as a liaison to the advisory council.

   d. The coordinator may employ professional, technical, research and clerical staff as necessary within the limits of available appropriations.

The provisions of Title 11A of the New Jersey Statutes shall apply to all personnel so employed.

e. The coordinator may solicit and accept grants of funds from the federal government and from other public and private sources.

4. The EMSC program shall include, but not be limited to, the establishment of the following:

a. Initial and continuing education programs for emergency medical services personnel that include training in emergency care of infants and children;

b. Guidelines for referring children to the appropriate emergency treatment facility;

c. Pediatric equipment guidelines for prehospital care;

d. Guidelines for hospital-based emergency departments appropriate for pediatric care to assess, stabilize, and treat critically ill infants and children, either to resolve the problem or to prepare the child for transfer to a pediatric intensive care unit or a pediatric trauma center;

e. Guidelines for pediatric intensive care units, pediatric trauma centers and intermediate care units fully equipped and staffed by appropriately trained critical care pediatric physicians, surgeons, nurses and therapists;

f. An interhospital transfer system for critically ill or injured children; and

g. Pediatric rehabilitation units staffed by rehabilitation specialists and capable of providing any service required to assure maximum recovery from the physical, emotional, and cognitive effects of critical illness and severe trauma.

5. a. There is created an Emergency Medical Services for Children Advisory Council to advise the Office of Emergency Medical Services and the coordinator of the EMSC program on all matters concerning emergency medical services for children. The advisory council shall assist in the formulation of policy and regulations to effectuate the purposes of this act.

b. The advisory council shall consist of a minimum of 12 public members to be appointed by the Governor, with the advice and consent of the Senate, for a term of three years. Membership of the advisory council shall include: one practicing pediatrician, one pediatric critical care physician and one pediatric physiatrist, to be appointed upon the recommendation of the New Jersey chapter of the American Academy of Pediatrics; one pediatric surgeon, to be appointed upon the recommendation of the New Jersey chapter of the American College of Surgeons; one emergency physician to be appointed upon the recommendation of the New Jersey Chapter of the American College of Emergency Physicians; one emergency medical technician and one paramedic, to be appointed upon the recommendation of the New Jersey State First Aid Council; one family practice physician, to be appointed upon the recommendation of the New Jersey chapter of the Academy of Family Practice; one registered emergency nurse, to be appointed upon the recommendation of the New Jersey State Nurses Association; and three members, each with a nonmedical background, two of whom are parents with children under the age of 18, to be appointed upon the joint recommendation of the Association for Children of New Jersey and the Junior Leagues of New Jersey.

c. Vacancies on the advisory council shall be filled for the unexpired term by appointment of the Governor in the same manner as originally filled. The members of the advisory council shall serve without compensation, but shall be reimbursed for necessary expenses incurred in the performance of their duties. The advisory council shall elect a chairperson, who may select from among the members a vice-chairperson and other officers or subcommittees which are deemed necessary or appropriate. The council may further organize itself in any manner it deems appropriate and enact bylaws as deemed necessary to carry out the responsibilities of the council.

6. The commissioner shall, pursuant to the "Administrative Procedure Act," P.L. 1968, c.410 (C.52:14B-1 et seq.), adopt rules and regulations necessary to effectuate the purposes of this act.

7. This act shall take effect immediately.

Statement

This bill establishes the Emergency Medical Services for Children program (EMSC) in the Office of Emergency Medical Services within the Department of Health. A full-time coordinator of the program shall be hired by the Commissioner of Health upon the recommendation of the Emergency Medical Services for Children Advisory Council established pursuant to section 5 of the bill.

The bill requires the coordinator to implement a statewide program of emergency medical services for children. The coordinator may employ necessary personnel, and solicit and accept grants of public and private funds. The EMSC program shall include, but not be limited to, establishment of the following:

1) Initial and continuing education programs for emergency medical services personnel that include training in the emergency care of infants and children;

2) Guidelines for referring children to the appropriate emergency treatment facility;

3) Pediatric equipment guidelines for prehospital care;

4) Guidelines for hospital-based emergency departments appropriate for pediatric care to assess, stabilize, and treat critically ill infants and children either to resolve the problem or to prepare the child for transfer to a pediatric intensive care unit or a pediatric trauma center;

5) Guidelines for pediatric intensive care units, pediatric trauma centers, and intermediate care units fully equipped and staffed by appropriately trained critical care pediatric physicians, surgeons, nurses and therapists;

6) An interhospital transfer system for critically ill or injured children; and

7) Pediatric rehabilitation units staffed by rehabilitation specialists and capable of providing any service required to assure maximum recovery from the physical, emotional, and cognitive effects of critical illness and severe trauma.

The commissioner is authorized, pursuant to the "Administrative Procedure Act," P.L. 1968, c.410 (C.52:14B-1 et seq.), to adopt rules and regulations necessary to effectuate the purposes of the bill.

Establishes Emergency Medical Services for Children Program.

INDEX

A

Abuse. *See* Child abuse and sexual
    assault
Access to emergency medical care,
    AAP Commission on Pediatric
    Emergency Medicine on, 90,
    177-79
Advanced Cardiac Life Support
    (course), 40
Advanced life support, minimum
    pediatric equipment and
    medications needed for, 51-52
Advanced Life Support (course), 19,
    35, 134
Advanced Pediatric Life Support
    (course), 6, 31-32, 40, 134, 156,
    161-62
Advanced Trauma Life Support
    (course), 40
Ambulance
  in interhospital transport, 70,
    71-72, 76-77, 78-80
  staffing of, 46-48
  in prehospital transport, 46-47
American Academy of Pediatrics
  advocacy role of, 121
  Committee on Child Abuse and
    Neglect, 104
  Committee on Pediatric emergency
    medicine, on access to
    emergency medical care, 90,
    177-79
  life support programs sponsored by,
    156-64
  on pediatrician's role in emergency
    medical services for children,
    125-27

American Association of Poison
    Control Centers, and
    certification of regional poison
    centers, 213-19
American College of Emergency
    Physicians
  advocacy role of, 121
  on basic life support equipment,
    50
  and development of disaster
    plans, 96
  sponsorship of Pediatric Life
    Support Class by, 156
American College of Surgeons
    Committee on Trauma
  and development of disaster
    plans, 96
  sponsorship of Advanced Trauma
    Life Support Class by, 40
American Heart Association
  sponsorship of Cardiac Life
    Support Class by, 40
  sponsorship of Pediatric Life
    Support Class by, 156
American Medical Association
  Commission on Emergency
    Medical Services, 13
      on pediatric emergencies,
        137-54
  Guidelines for the Categorization
    of Hospital Emergency
    Capabilities, 90
Anticipatory guidance, role of
    physician in, 20-28
Automobile, private, in interhospital
    transport, 70, 77

B

Basic life support
  minimum pediatric equipment
    and supplies needed for, 50
  minimum resuscitation equipment
    and supplies needed for the
    newborn, 52
Basic emergency medical technician
  (EMT), 45
Basic Life Support for Health Care
  Providers (course), 19, 134,
  156, 157-58

C

Child abuse and sexual assault, 65,
  101-4
  evaluation of, 66
  historical indicators of, 102
  laboratory and radiographic
    indicators of, 103
  medical diagnostic programs in US,
    and Canada, 192-212
  physical indicators of, 102
  sample data sheet for, 105-7
Child Abuse and Sexual Assault
  Centers, 101
Cluster suicide, 104
Communication, with referral
  hospital, 92-93
Community advocates, parent role as,
  28
Community hospital emergency
  departments, 55-68
  implementation models for
    standards, 66
  organization of, 57-59, 64-66
  standards for, 60-65
Consolidated Budget Reconciliation
  Act (COBRA) (1985), 72, 73, 74
Consultant/child advocate, primary
  care provider as, 6
Costs, transport, 91-92

CPR

  maintaining certification in, 40-41
  need for office staff knowledge
    in, 35

D

Deaths in the emergency department,
  110-14
Direct medical control, 12-13
Disaster management, role of
  physician in, 6
Disaster plan, 96-97
  JCAHO on, 114-15
Drug dosages, method for estimating
  weight in determining, 169-76

E

Educator, physician as, 5
Emergencies, 95, 134
  in physician's office, 39
  preparing parents to cope
    with, 19-29
  psychiatric, 104, 108
  true, 136
Emergency care
  documentation of, 41-43
  in-hospital, 13-14
Emergency care provider,
  physician as, 5-6
Emergency care site, physician's
  office as, 31-44
Emergency department. See also
  Community hospital
  emergency departments
  pediatric deaths in, 110-14
Emergency Department Approved
  for Pediatrics (EDAP), 56, 60,
  65, 134
  standards for, 60-64
Emergency Medical Services Act
  (1973), 11-12
  specialty referral component
    of the, 11

Emergency Medical Service (EMS)
    system, 9-11
    access and system entry, 12
    community hospital as a
        component of, 55-67
    definitive care, 14-15
    in-hospital emergency care, 13-14
    prehospital care, 12-13
    rehabilitation, 15-16
Emergency Medical Services for
    Children (EMS-C), 9, 134
    advocating for, 117-22
    components of a comprehensive, 3-4
    referral hospital as component of,
        89-94
    role of primary care physician in,
        1-7, 9-18
    specific objectives of, 125
Emergency Medical Services for
    Children Innovation Bank, 121
Emergency Medical Services for
    Children products, 130-33
Emergency Medical Services-C
    (EMS-C) Project
    contact personnel, 128-29
    goals of, 15
Emergency medical
    technician-ambulance
        (EMT-A), 47
Emergency medical technician-basic
        (EMT), 135
Emergency medical
    technician-paramedic (EMT-P),
        45, 135
Emergency medicine, as specialty, 58
Emergent, 96, 135, 138
EMT-2, 47
Enhanced 911 system, 10, 12
Equipment
    for advanced and basic life support,
        50-52
    emergency, in physician's office,
        37-39
    in prehospital transport, 49

F
Field triage, 13
First aid
    parent role in, 26-27
    suggested supplies for, 27
First responders, 46-48
    training for, 46-48

G
Guidelines for the Categorization of
    Hospital Emergency
    Capabilities (AMA), 90

H
Helicopter, in interhospital transport,
    70, 80-82
High-risk children, parent role with,
    28-29
Hospital
    receiving, 75-76
    referral, 89-94

I
ICD-E coding systems, 20
ICD-H coding systems, 20
Indirect medical control, 12, 48
In-hospital emergency care, 13-14
Injury Control, 22
Interhospital transport, 71-87, 137
    advance preparation, 71-72
    ambulance, 72, 73-74, 78-80
    COBRA/OBRA legislation on, 72-75
    communication with the receiving
        hospital, 75-76
    follow-up, 86
    options for, 76-84
    private automobile, 70, 77
    transport teams, 80-86
International Class of Disease-E
    coding (ICD-E), 20
International Class of Disease-H
    coding (ICD-H), 20

Pediatric age group, rapid method for estimating weight and resuscitation drug dosages from length in the, 169-76
Pediatric Basic Life Support (course), 156, 158-59
Pediatric Critical Care Center (PCC), 56, 65, 136
Pediatric emergencies, AMA Commission on Emergency Medical Services on, 137-54
Pediatric emergency medicine, as specialty, 58
Pediatric reference library, 58, 165-68
Pediatric Resuscitation Measuring Tape, 43
Personnel, in prehospital transport, 46-48
Physician skills, in emergency care, 39-40
Poison centers, 108-9
    certified regional, 213-19
Prehospital care, 12-13
Prehospital transport, 72, 136
    equipment, 49
    medical control, 48-49
    personnel in, 46-48
    triage, 48
    of your patient, 45-51
Prevention, parent role in, 20-22
Psychiatric emergencies, 104, 106, 108, 110

Q

Quality assurance programs, for the emergency department, 111, 114

R

Receiving hospital, communication with, 75-76
Recognition/access, parent role in, 22-26

Record-keeping, importance of, 41-43
Referral hospital, 89-94
    choice of, 90
    communication with, 92-93
    criteria for referral/acceptance, 92
    responsibilities of, 91
    reverse referral, 93
    transfer agreements, 90-91
    transport costs, 91-92
Referring physician, communication with receiving hospital, 75-76
Rural Emergency Departments Approved for Pediatrics, 65
Rural settings, victims of trauma in, 14-15

S

Secondary transport, 70, 136
Sexual abuse. See Child abuse and sexual assault
SIDs. See Sudden infant death syndrome (SIDS)
Special situation planning, 95-116
    child abuse and sexual assault, 101-4
        sample data sheet for, 105-7
    deaths in the emergency department, 110-14
    mass casualty/disaster plan, 96-97
    poisoning-poison control centers, 108-9
    sudden infant death syndrome (SIDS), 109-10, 220-50
    suicide and psychiatric emergencies, 104, 108
    unaccompanied minor requiring care, 98-101
Staff preparation, for handling emergencies, 35-36
Stand-by Emergency Department Approved for Pediatrics, 65
Sudden illness and injury, characteristics of, 10

Sudden infant death syndrome
(SIDS), 109-10
centers for, 220-50
Suicide
cluster, 104
and psychiatric emergencies, 104,
108

T

Telephone triage, 47-48
TIPP program, 21
Transfer agreement, 89, 90-91, 137
sample, 183-85
Transfer decision, 91
Transport
interhospital, 70
prehospital, 70
secondary, 70

Transport teams, 80-82
dedicated pediatric or neonatal,
82-84
preparing for arrival of, 84-86
Trauma center, 13
Triage, 33-35, 57
field, 13
in prehospital transport, 48
telephone, 47-48
Triage log, 97
Triage officer, physician as, 5
Triage tag, 97
True emergency, 96, 136

U

Urgent, 96, 136

W

Weight method for estimating for
drug dosages, 169-76